There's Much More Than A Smile

There's Much More Than A Smile

✦

What You Should Know About Caring For Your Teeth

Brent T. Clifford

Writers Club Press
New York Lincoln Shanghai

There's Much More Than A Smile
What You Should Know About Caring For Your Teeth

Writers Club Press
an imprint of iUniverse, Inc.

For information address:
iUniverse, Inc.
2021 Pine Lake Road, Suite 100
Lincoln, NE 68512
www.iuniverse.com

General information only, consult your Dentist before starting any new method of home care. Library of Congress Catalog Card Number: TX 5-638-476

ISBN: 0-595-21699-4

Printed in the United States of America

Contents

FOREWORD

Once in awhile as we listen to the news on the radio and television, we are informed by some major health care organization that the most prevalent disease in the world is not AIDS, Cancer or Heart Problems, it is Tooth Decay. Why, with all our advancements in medicine, is tooth decay still the leading disease in the world and even in our more advanced countries? I have observed that it is caused by an attitude and a lack of education. We have the attitude that decay is acceptable, that everyone has it and it is natural. We have the attitude that my parents and grandparents had dentures and it is acceptable for me to have dentures also. We do not believe that we can do much to prevent decay and accept it as a natural consequence. We are raised already defeated, because we have adapted to the loss of our teeth and do not recognize it as a major loss. We as a whole do not know how to correctly take care of our teeth and maintain them and yet it is so basic to our good health.

There is a way to stop decay from affecting everyone's life, and that is education. The more we know the less it will affect us and our families. It is with this purpose in mind that I have written this book. In writing this book I have drawn from over 20 years experience in dentistry, however, I am not a dentist. I was trained by the U.S. AIR FORCE to be a dental assistant, a dental hygienist, and an expanded functions assistant. I have worked with over 80 different dentists. Part of what I have learned I am passing on to you. Many of you do not know how to correctly take care of your teeth, or the consequences of what is happening to your teeth. This book will give you some basic guidance and insight necessary to help you. It is not intended to be all-inclusive or tell you everything that can happen. You will not need a background in dentistry to understand what I have written. It is writ-

ten in a very basic way and in a language that should be easily under-
stood. I have written in this book, what I would tell you if you were a
patient and asking me questions. I have left out most of the dental
terms and substituted words, which are more common so that you may
understand what I am trying to say. It will inform you about many
things you can and should be aware of. It will let you know something
about the things you will encounter in your life. I hope you not only
learn from this book, but enjoy reading it as well.

WHY WRITE THIS BOOK?

Why am I writing this book? During my over twenty years experience in dentistry, I have been amazed at the lack of knowledge people have about their teeth. Then I look back on how I was raised and realize why. First of all, my parents never knew anything about how to care for their teeth. They were both plagued with dental problems and ended up with dentures. In school I was taught only to brush my teeth and even then I was taught incorrectly. Everything else I learned from the advertisements for different dental products. Although that left me with many questions about which product was really the best. The very few articles written about dental problems which I read by chance, I usually didn't think would ever apply to me. When I visited my dentist (which was only when I had a problem) I did not spend a lot of time asking him question, I just wanted him to fix my problem and let me out of there. Like most of you, I did not like being there. Do you recognize any of my reasons for not knowing more? Have you had the same experience?

I have talked with many people who just like me did not know how to take care of their teeth and in many, many cases were taught the wrong things (like I was) and have paid a big price in the loss of their teeth. In most cases they also paid a big price in dollars. **This does not need to happen**! This is part of the reason I decided to write this book. To help inform those who want to be informed. Many people want to take care of their teeth but have been given no information or given the wrong information. They will never get their dental condition completely under control until they get the right information. It is my intent that this book will be a good place for you to start.

Does this book contain all the information necessary, No! It is very important that you understand that what I have written in this book is my own ideas taken from the experiences I have had with those dentists I have worked with. It is not intended to replace appropriate dental advice and treatment from your dentist who knows you and can evaluate your needs. I do not know all the information necessary for every problem there is which will involve the mouth. Your dentist is still the best one to seek out for information. I want to give you enough information so you will be able to ask good questions and know which direction you should be going in and then recognize it when you hear it. **Most of your dental problems will be created and controlled by you. You can have what ever you are willing to work for, that's the bottom line.**

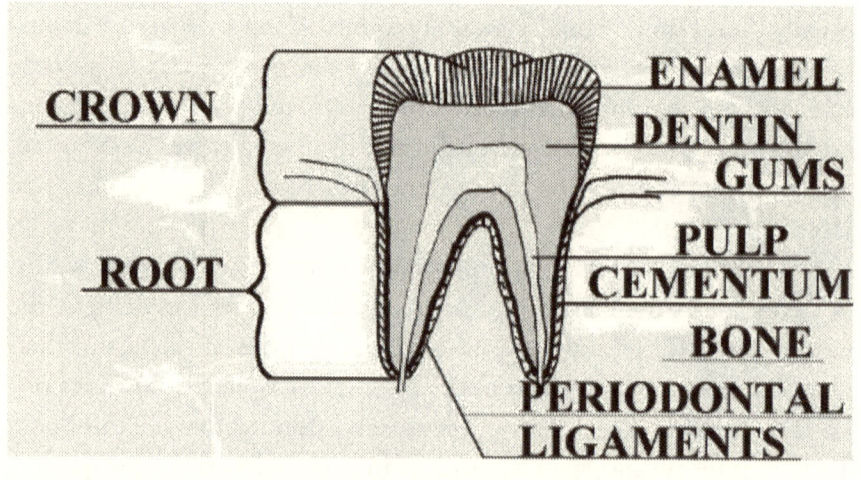

Anatomy of a tooth and surrounding tissues. (Refer to this illustration as you read this book.)

INFECTION CONTROL

This subject is getting a lot of publicity and is in the forefront of dentistry. Almost every dental publication will have an update on infection control. The dentists themselves well be aware of what is current.

With the concern about contagious diseases, especially AIDS and Hepatitis, cleanliness is a necessity. Besides cleanliness, there are what is called barrier techniques and infection control. For those who have no idea what that is, it is doing everything necessary to prevent the spread of infectious disease and the bacteria or viruses that cause them. This has been helped by OSHA (Occupational Safety and Health Administration). As of 1992, OSHA has put requirements on the dental profession for infection control. Many of the requirements will affect only the dentists and their staff, but some will affect you as patients. As a minimum, the dentists and their treatment staff must wear examination gloves, facemasks, protective eyewear, and fluid resistant gowns. Some dentists will go farther by wearing a second pair of gloves, and a face shield.

There are many styles of gowns worn, and no particular style is dictated, although some are recommended. The recommendation is a gown with a high neck, long sleeves with cuffs, and long enough to go below the knees. Another reason for the dentists and their assistants to wear so much protective gear is if they have anything, be it only a cold or sore throat. You do not need it, and it helps protect you.

If you feel your dentist is not doing the minimum requirements, you may want to reconsider letting them work on you. If they are not following this portion of the requirements, what are they doing about the rest? Some of the other requirements are; instruments that are used in your mouth must be sterilized in a heat or heat-pressure sterilizer, not a liquid. My preference is the instruments are bagged as well unless they are kept in a separate room until needed. I also prefer the instruments not be taken out of their bags until I am seated in the room, so I can see that sterilization is being done.

When I first started working in dentistry, all we did was wipe the hand pieces and instruments off with alcohol and use them again. We cannot do that now, not with the possibility of AIDS and Hepatitis as great as it is. Hand pieces are made to be and must be sterilized. If the hand pieces are cleaned according to the manufacturers' instructions, they should be OK. If you are worried about whether the hand piece has been cleaned well enough because of what is called suck-back, ask your dentist. Dental units made since 1985 have a one-way valve that prevents suck-back. Those made prior to that time can have a one-way valve installed, which prevents suck-back. Most dentists should have this problem taken care of, but ask anyway. It's you in the chair.

Additional things you need to be aware of are cross contamination and barrier techniques. This means if the dentist is working on you and they have to touch something else, (be it supplies, equipment, telephone, pencils, whatever). They take their gloves off, throw them away and put on a clean pair when they start working on you again. They may wear over gloves, which they put on over their gloves, do what they were going to do and take them off before they return to work on you. The bottom line is the dentist does not put gloves into your mouth that have touched anything that may be contaminated by someone else.

The equipment must be cleaned between each patient. You may have a dentist that has his or her equipment covered with plastic, which is changed between each patient. The plastic can reduce the cleaning time because it is discarded. If not, the equipment needs to be cleaned and sprayed with a disinfectant. These disinfectants require a 1 to 10 minute wait to disinfect, and then they need to dry or be wiped dry. If you see a patient come out of a room and you go right in, unless it's covered with plastic, it may not be disinfected. Do not be afraid to ask your dentist if they are disinfecting the treatment rooms between patients.

Why am I big on infection control? I know how easily bacteria and viruses can be spread. Each time the dentists use their high-speed hand piece, they are shooting an aerosol that contains bacteria and viruses from 5 to 7 feet into the air. This does not stay in the air, it lands everywhere. Each time they touch something new they spread germs. You have no idea what the patients before you may have had, and you should expect the dentist to protect you the best they can.

BRUSHING YOUR TEETH

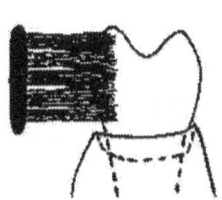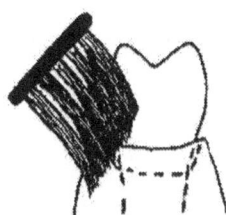

Holding your toothbrush flat against your teeth will only allow you to clean your teeth and not the area below the gum line. Holding your toothbrush at a 45-degree angle you will brush your teeth, and get the bristles under the gum line and clean the sulcus. You will massage the gum tissue at the same time. The results are healthier teeth and gums.

This is one of the most important parts of this book, so please read it carefully. **Brushing your teeth is the heart of good oral hygiene. It is the single most important thing you can do to protect your teeth, gums and overall oral health.**

I know you have heard this, "Be sure to brush your teeth after every meal and whenever you eat anything." We have been taught this by our parents, teachers, dentists, and everyone else. If you have developed a habit of brushing three times a day, do not stop. If you have not, do not feel guilty or that you are a bad parent if your children don't. In my opinion, it is not necessary! Now don't stop reading here, hear me out! I am going to tell you some things you may have never heard before.

Why do we brush? We brush to remove food particles and bacteria. Food particles and bacteria are the causes of; plaque, tartar, decay, gum disease, periodontal disease and of course **Bad Breath**. There are other things that contribute too, but I'll stay with the things you are acquainted with.

When we eat, we coat our teeth with food particles. They combine with bacteria and saliva in our mouth and form plaque. It is plaque that is the cause of our dental problems. Plaque is a soft, sticky substance that adheres to our teeth. When left on our teeth for over twenty-four hours, it starts to harden and forms tartar (Calculus). It attacks our teeth and gums and starts its destructive process. If it is removed during this twenty-four hour period, the cycle is stopped and must be started over. Therefore, in my opinion, it is only necessary to brush at least once a day. However, your brushing must be completely effective.

Most of us will usually not do an effective job of brushing if we are brushing for only 1 to 3 minutes a day. If that is how long you brush, you probably have dental problems. Most of us need to spend more time just brushing. The reason is we must be thorough, and that takes time. The makers of dental products are trying to get you to brush more effectively in those 1 to 3 minutes rather than brush longer. That is the reasoning behind many of the mechanical devices and that is good for those who use these devices. But what about those who only use a regular toothbrush? If you brush effectively in those 1 to 3 minutes, keep at it, but if not, the best thing to do may be to increase the amount of time you spend brushing.

The best time to brush is before you go to bed. Think about it. If you brush only in the morning, the food particles and bacteria are on your teeth for approximately 24 hours. If you brush before bed, these same particles are only on your teeth from when you eat in the morning until you brush. This lessens the opportunity for dental problems.

Most of us do not want to stand at a sink for 10 to 20 minutes brushing our teeth, and we will not develop a habit of doing this. This is what I do and recommend. I brush (without toothpaste) while watching TV, reading a book, doing homework, and when working at my computer. I do not do it when in a restaurant, or working. I have done this for years and although I've had a lot of dental work because of neglect while I was young, I haven't had any new problems of any sort for the past 26 years. I have not had any new decay, and my gums do not bleed and are in excellent shape.

When I brush this way, I swallow my saliva. I swallow it all day long, so it's not any different. You just have to get use to it. I take the time to brush each tooth and spend the time necessary to get it clean. I do it unconsciously because I'm doing other things and I don't rush through it. My teeth really do feel clean when I'm finished. Another advantage I received, is that brushing my teeth helped me to stay awake and alert. It may do the same for you.

Although I do not use toothpaste at the above mentioned times, I still rinse my toothbrush each time I finish. If I did not rinse my toothbrush, then I'm going to use a toothbrush that will have food debris and bacteria (which has been growing since last use), and reintroduce it into my mouth. That's a way of causing new problems. Always rinse your toothbrush.

Spending a lot of time brushing will do you more good if you are brushing correctly. When I was a child, they taught me to hold my toothbrush flat against my teeth and sweep it towards the top or biting surface of my teeth. I did this for almost twenty years. Twenty years of brushing incorrectly, and I have the fillings to prove it. I also had problems with my gums bleeding. I was 25 years of age before I was correctly taught to take care of my teeth.

Let me give you some ideas on brushing correctly. Hold your soft bristled toothbrush at an angle (about 45 degrees) so the bristles will go underneath your gum tissue. You have a small open area around each tooth, next to the gum line. It is called the sulcus. This is where debris and bacteria stay and begin their damage. Use a gentle back and forth motion or a circular motion. You want to get the bristles of your toothbrush under your gum tissue so it can remove the bacteria and debris. This will also remove any plaque, all in one motion. Take time to clean as much of the area between your teeth as your toothbrush will reach.

Do this on all your teeth, front, back, on top, and behind your back teeth.

The areas of your mouth that plaque turns into tartar the most, are on the outside of your top molars and the inside of your lower front teeth. It does this because these are the areas where saliva enters your mouth and mixes with plaque to form tartar. Because of this fact, you should spend more time brushing these areas.

If you are not sure you are doing a thorough job of brushing, try using a disclosing tablet. It is what your dentist or hygienist has you chew up and then spit out to show where you are missing with your toothbrush. You can purchase them at your drugstore or market. If you are trying to get younger children to brush correctly, they are a great help. Be careful when you have them spit. They can spit it all over and it can be a mess to clean.

If your gum tissue is unhealthy, it may bleed for a while when you begin brushing this way (see the section on bleeding gums). After you have brushed correctly for several weeks, you will notice your teeth and gums feel better, and the bleeding should be stopped. If the bleeding has not stopped, see your dentist. You may need additional help.

If you have difficulty brushing your teeth and getting under your gums as well, you may want to concentrate on doing each one separately, until you can do it automatically. The important thing is that each area must be cleaned daily. It does not matter what type of brush stroke you use, just that you clean each area thoroughly.

FLOSSING

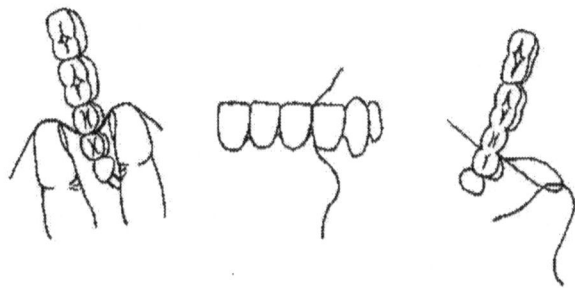

If your teeth are close together, you cannot get your toothbrush through the contacts. You must use dental floss if you want to clean these areas. Wrap your floss around your middle finger (or two fingers) and leave yourself about 1 inch between your fingers to floss with. Push the floss back, away from, the area you are flossing. This will allow the floss to slide into the sulcus and not cut your gum tissue. Your floss will go below your gum tissue and not hurt you. If you take it down to far, you could cause some pain and damage so be careful. By using a floss threader, you can get the floss under your bridge. It is vital these teeth be flossed as well as all others.

The purpose of dental floss is very misunderstood. It is one of the reasons I decided to write this book. Dental floss is not something to use only when you get something caught between your teeth, or when you need extra strong string. Although it does have many uses, it is designed to remove food and plaque from between your teeth and below your gum tissue. It, along with brushing properly, is the most important thing you can do to keep your teeth and gums healthy. We would tell our patients that they only had to floss the teeth they wanted to keep.

The value of flossing should not be overlooked. We are all aware of the importance of brushing our teeth. Our parents, teachers, dentist, and the mass media have drilled it into us. However, little is said about flossing, and yet, it is as important as brushing, if not more so. The value of flossing has not been stressed enough. If you get your teeth cleaned by a hygienist, they may tell you to floss your teeth and hopefully, what will happen if you do not.

Often, no one gives you the big picture of why it is so necessary. When you brush your teeth, you brush 3 sides of your teeth: the front, back, and top. But what about between your teeth? There are still 2 surfaces, which for most of us, our toothbrushes will not reach very well. It is vital that these surfaces be cleaned as well. Many of our cavities start between the teeth where the toothbrush will not reach. Floss will, and it will clean effectively if done correctly.

Fighting tooth decay is not the reason I feel so strongly about flossing. The reason is periodontal disease. I have seen people with beautiful teeth and no decay, lose those teeth. The reason is periodontal disease. It is believed by many people, my parents lost their teeth when they were young (between 30 and 45) and I will as well. That may be the case, but it does not have to be. In most cases, you can keep your teeth throughout your life, if you keep them clean, and it takes more than just brushing.

Let me explain. As we eat and drink, there are tiny particles that are trapped between our teeth and under our gums. If they are not removed daily, they begin to form plaque that attacks our tooth structure and gums. As it attacks our gum tissue, our gums may get infected or very red and bleed easily when brushed. You may get puss coming from some areas. There may be tenderness and slight swelling. These are the first signs of gum disease or periodontal disease. It is nothing to be upset about. If you catch it right away and start brushing, flossing correctly and rinsing your mouth with warm saltwater, you will stop it yourself in a couple of weeks. I should say you can stop the symptoms. You should still have a dentist check you over and have your gums and bone condition evaluated. The condition of gum disease will be discussed more in the section on periodontal disease.

Before I go any further, let me help you decide which type of floss you may want, or should be using. If you are a beginner at using floss, I recommend that you use waxed floss. There is less chance you will damage your gum tissue while you are learning to maneuver your fingers inside your mouth. Waxed floss does give off a small wax residue. It is not harmful and you will probably not notice it. If you have teeth that are close together, waxed floss is best because it will slide through the contacts points better than the non-waxed floss. When you get more adept at using floss, you may want to switch to a non-waxed floss, it tends to clean better.

Floss comes in different sizes. There is a fine non-waxed floss (which can be used between teeth that are close together), medium sized floss, and what is called dental tape, or wide waxed floss. If you have an advanced periodontal condition or large spaces between your teeth, you may want to try using what is called dental ribbon. It is floss with a yarn attached. It has the advantage of covering, and in fact polishing, a large area very quickly. It should only be used when there is a wide space between the teeth.

There are several methods for using floss, but I will give you the one I find works best. Because you will be placing your fingers in your mouth, I recommend you wash your hands before you start. Take a piece of floss about 24 inches long and wrap it around your two middle fingers, leaving your index fingers free. I recommend using two fingers instead of one so it does not cut off your blood circulation so much. Keep an eye on your fingertips and if they are turning blue, loosen your floss. Wrap it about two times, enough to keep the floss from sliding free. Wrap the remainder of the floss around the two middle fingers on the other hand. Let out enough floss that you can hold it by applying pressure against it with your index fingers and your thumbs, and have about 1 inch between them (refer to the illustration). As you use the floss you will unwrap it from one hand and wrap it up on the other, thus giving yourself fresh floss when you want it.

Sometimes it is easier to use a mirror when you begin flossing, but you should work at being able to do it without a mirror. You will have to put your fingers inside your mouth to floss correctly, and you will use your index fingers and thumbs together, depending on which teeth you are flossing.

Begin by gently sliding the floss between your teeth. Do not snap it between your teeth because you could damage your gum tissue. After you have the floss between your teeth, put your fingers back, or away from the tooth you are flossing. The floss will wrap around the tooth surface you want to floss (refer to the illustration). Gently move the floss up and down several times, or until the tooth feels clean. It may take some time before you will feel the difference, but it will come. Be sure to take the floss below the gums next to the tooth. There is space there where the gums are unattached to the teeth. It is vital this area be cleaned, and is in fact one of the main reasons you should floss your teeth. Take the floss as far down as you can without hurting your gums. Do this with every tooth. Do it on teeth that do not have an adjacent tooth next to them and behind your back teeth.

When you are flossing and getting your floss under the gum tissue as you should, you may not be able to get it back up. You may have very tight contacts, a filling between your teeth with an overhang on it, or perhaps you have a crown that the margins hang over a little. It is important that you do not try to pull your floss back up through the contacts. You could pull your crown off, dislodge your filling, or break off your floss between your teeth and not be able to get it out. If you break it off, try using another piece of waxed floss and if you get it through, do not pull it back up. What you do in all cases is release the floss from one of your hands and pull it out, not up. However, keep flossing those areas, they will need it even more than other areas. If you get it stuck and cannot dislodge it with your floss, see your dentist and let them dislodge it, do not try everything you can think of. You could do a lot of damage.

If you are unable to use your fingers inside your mouth, do not give up. There are floss aids, which will do the job for you, and they work very effectively. They are very good if you are flossing the teeth of someone else, such as an elderly or handicapped person, or younger children. These people need their teeth flossed as much as you do and it will save you a lot of dental bills if you take the time to do it. Teach them to do it if possible.

If you have a bridge in your mouth, you must floss under it. What will happen if you do not is you will develop periodontal disease under that bridge, and in time you will lose that bridge and possibly your teeth as well. It can be avoided and maintained very easily with the use of a device called a floss threader. There are several types made from plastic and wire. They operate by the same principle as a needle and thread. You thread the floss through the end of the floss threader and then run the floss threader under your bridge. Take and floss the teeth at both ends of your bridge and run it along the bridge as well to remove any buildup it may have. It is a simple thing to do, but can have some very bad effects if not done.

I am asked when is the best time to floss and how often. How often, is daily. The best time is when you can fit it in and make it a habit. You will want about 5 minutes after you become proficient. I recommend doing it at night before going to bed. Do it when brushing your teeth. Not everyone will have the same schedule, but do it sometime during the day.

Remember, I said it is best to use a mirror when you start learning to floss. When you can, stop using the mirror. This will allow you the freedom of being able to floss somewhere other than in your bathroom. My best time to floss is when I am watching TV, reading or working at my computer. I am not limited in time and I can do as thorough a flossing as I want to. The important thing is that you floss your teeth daily. If you cannot do it for five minutes, do it for as long as you can, but do it!

TOOTHBRUSHES

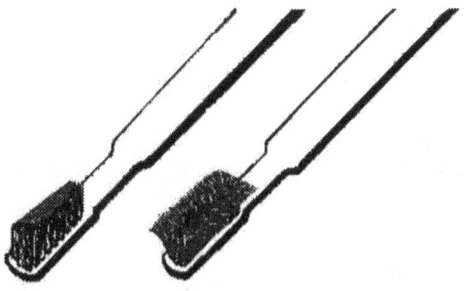

A toothbrush is the most important instrument for proper oral hygiene. The size and shape are not as important as that it has soft bristles and it is used regularly. When your brush begins to flare out, it is time to replace it with a new brush.

As you might expect, I have definite ideas about what type of toothbrush is best. When I was young, I would only buy hard toothbrushes. I liked the fact I could get one to last for almost a year. I also felt that I was getting my teeth very clean because the bristles were so stiff. Well, thank goodness I learned differently. The only toothbrush I will use and recommend is a soft toothbrush. Hard and medium toothbrushes have their place, if you like them, use them. For me they are great for cleaning the tile in the bathroom or around the windows, or similar things. They do not have the flexibility to get between your teeth and under your gum tissue. This is part of the reason people end up with gum disease. They will also tear up your gum tissue. If you look in a mirror and see stains between your teeth where a hard or medium toothbrush cannot reach, you can easily tell that your brush, or the way you use it, is not doing all it should. You need to check your brush and the method you use. You should be able to keep your teeth free from stains if you're brushing correctly.

The style of toothbrush you use is not as vital as that it has soft bristles. If you like a straight one or one with the bent head or any of the new combinations, it doesn't matter. All of them should work as designed. What matters is that you feel comfortable with what you use, and use it often. I do have my favorite brand, and although I try many of the new styles, I still prefer one brand.

Change toothbrushes about every 3 months. If you notice the bristles on your toothbrush have started to fan out, it is time to change. Watch your children's toothbrushes as well and change them when needed.

If you are using a hard or medium toothbrush, you may not think you are cleaning your teeth when you switch to a soft brush. Keep with it and you should notice a big difference before too long. Most likely, like me, you will never go back to the hard or medium brush.

It is important that you keep your toothbrush clean, rinse it after each use. Store it in an area that it can be kept separate from other toothbrushes, especially if anyone is sick. Most people do not think about this, but if your toothbrush is kept in a bathroom, it is advised that it be kept as far away as possible from your toilet because of the aerosol that is created each time the toilet is flushed.

MECHANICAL TOOTHBRUSHES AND IRRIGATION DEVICES

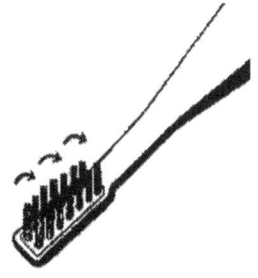

A rotary type of mechanical toothbrush is suggested because it will allow you to clean under the gum tissue better than one, which goes up and down.

I am sold on brushing your teeth, using a good toothbrush and spending the time to do the job right. What about powered toothbrushes? I have some concerns about using them, let me explain. The toothbrushes do what they are designed to do, it's the user I have the concern about. Often, when a person uses a powered toothbrush, they do not take the time to do a thorough job of brushing. As stated in other places of this book, a study shows in our country, we spend an average of three minutes brushing our teeth. Using a powered toothbrush may make three minutes more effective, if you will take the time. Yet, as in most things we do, we tend to take shortcuts and if you skimp on using even a powered brush, you may have the security of thinking you are doing enough, when you may not be. I have some concerns with that and you should to!

Another reason is if your powered toothbrush is weak or out completely, you won't brush effectively and spend the time needed. If your children use only the powered toothbrush, and do not know how to effectively clean their teeth with a regular toothbrush, you could be creating long-range problems for them and yourself.

I wholeheartedly support using a powered toothbrush by those who have a disability or handicap that prevents them from using a regular toothbrush. It's the best thing to do. They need extra attention paid to their oral hygiene.

If you use a powered toothbrush, I suggest one that rotates the bristles. This is so you can clean under the gums as effectively as possible. Also, get brushes with soft bristles. If your teeth start to show signs of sensitivity, ease up on your pressure, and use less toothpaste. You may have to even go back to your regular toothbrush for a while, and do not be as aggressive when you use your powered brush again.

How about water irrigation devices? They are great for the patient with deep periodontal pockets. Be careful you do not turn the pressure to high, you can damage the periodontal ligaments if you do. For the rest of us they are OK if, and I repeat if, you are not using them as a substitute for brushing and flossing. They will not clean as well. It's like washing your dirty car with only a power sprayer. It removes most of the dirt, but doesn't clean the car as well as washing it with a cloth and soapy water. What can I say!

DECAY OR CAVITIES

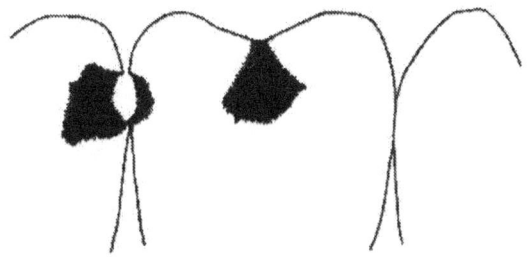

The decayed area of your tooth may look very small to you, but it can be very large. Have your teeth checked by a dentist yearly.

The most widely spread diseases of mankind is dental decay. It is also one of the easiest to prevent (refer to the sections on brushing and flossing). So you will understand more about decay and how it affects you, let me tell you briefly how it develops.

It is caused by plaque on your teeth. Underneath the plaque, bacteria are trapped and they form with carbohydrates from your food. This ferments and produces acid, which is trapped and protected by the plaque. This acid attacks the enamel on your teeth. This is known as decalcification and you may first notice it as an area on your teeth that looks chalky. If you begin taking care of it at this point you can still stop it. If it has entered into the enamel, but not into the dentin, it is known as incipient decay. It is the one your dentist tells the assistant to write "watch" next to, when you have an exam. If you keep it clean, you can slow it down and even stop it at that point. If you don't, it will break through the enamel and become full blown decay. Once decay has broken through the enamel, it will spread through the dentin quickly. This is because your dentin is not as hard as your enamel. If left alone, it can take months or years before it will reach the point you will lose your tooth. That all depends on how well you take care of your teeth.

Decay will usually start between your teeth and on the top of your back teeth. If you leave plaque on your teeth near the gum line, then you'll also get decay in that area as well. Decay can be misleading because you may see a small hole on the surface of the tooth, however below the surface the decay will mushroom or spread out. It will do this because the dentin is much softer than enamel and there is nothing to stop it from doing its destruction.

Once your enamel has decayed, it is gone and you cannot get it back. At best, you will get it restored by a good dentist. That tooth is now affected for the rest of your life. Please re-read the section on brushing and flossing. Decay is so easy to prevent.

TEMPORARY FILLINGS

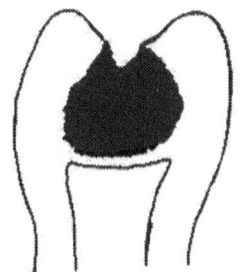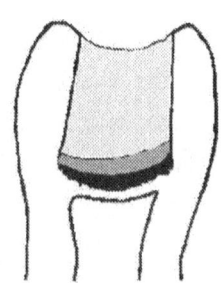

When you have large decay, talk with your dentist about the options before you begin treatment. If you take an interest and show you know something about what is going on, you are more likely to get the treatment you want. An option to consider is to remove most of the decay (all the decay if possible), then place a base of calcium hydroxide, and a temporary filling. Left for about six months, many teeth can be saved from root canals or extraction.

There are times your dentist will want you to have a temporary filling. Let me help you understand what you are getting and why.

One type of temporary filling is not used as much as it could be, but it is an alternative you should be aware of. When your dentist is working on your teeth and removing decay, they may get very close to the nerve (pulp chamber). They may tell you that you now need a root canal or an extraction. Well, let me tell you about an indirect pulp cap and a direct pulp cap.

All the decay does not necessarily have to be removed. If they stop just short of exposing the nerve, put a base material of calcium hydroxide over the nerve and a temporary filling over that. Leave it for 6 months. They can sometimes save that tooth and not need a root canal or extraction. This is called an indirect pulp cap.

If they remove the decay and expose the nerve (pulp chamber), they can still cover the opening, if small enough, with calcium hydroxide and a temporary filling. Leave it for 6 months. This will also save the tooth sometimes. This is called a direct pulp cap because the pulp is exposed.

The reason this works is the calcium hydroxide causes a secondary growth of dentin over the nerve. Many times this will grow thick enough in 6 months to allow the dentist to then remove all the decay and put in a permanent filling or crown if needed. This is a good option if conditions are right. You do run some risk because you do not know how that tooth will react once you leave the dental office. You could have it abscess (read section on an abscess). If you elect to have it done, request it in advance of the dentist working on you so they know you want to try it.

You have to treat a temporary filling with extreme care. You cannot chew anything hard on it, you may cause too much trauma to the nerve, or the temporary may break out. You must continue to brush and floss it, but be careful so that you don't dislodge it. Perhaps have your dentist take the tooth slightly out of occlusion so you don't bite so hard on it. The older you are, the less chance you have this will work for you. If you are middle aged or older, you will not grow secondary dentin as fast, if at all. However, if you are in good health and want to try it, go for it. You may be successful. This procedure also runs the risk of sealing off your pulp canals, making it harder, if not impossible, to have a root canal done later. Be aware there are risks with this procedure.

Sometimes temporary fillings are used to calm down a tooth that is very sensitive. Some temporary filling materials contain eugenol that has a sedative effect on your teeth. It can take awhile, but it can help save your tooth and prevent more extensive work. Request this type of filling if you want to try either the indirect or direct pulp cap.

Sometimes temporary fillings are placed when many teeth are badly decayed. The dentist may remove all the decay on several teeth, knowing they will not have the time to fill them with permanent restorations. They do this to get the decay out and stop it from further destroying your teeth. Once they get all the decay out, they put the temporary fillings in and later, they will place fillings or what ever is required. The important thing is you must return and have the work completed. Temporaries are just that, temporary. They will not last forever.

Another time a temporary filling is used is when the dentist is not sure if the tooth will abscess or not. They place a temporary, perhaps give you some antibiotics and have you wait a while for additional treatment. If the tooth survives, a filling is placed. If not, a root canal or extraction is done.

Temporary fillings may also be in the form of a stainless steel, plastic or aluminum crown. These are placed over a tooth that is badly broken down or has been prepared for a crown. This type is designed to protect your tooth from breaking down. A word of caution about this type of temporary crown; they often have large overhangs which trap debris and bacteria. This can lead to gum problems, so be sure you brush and floss around them. When you floss, **pull your floss out, not up/down**. Be sure to return to your dentist as soon as possible and have the temporary crown removed and replaced with a more permanent restoration or crown.

There are different types of filling materials used as temporaries. Each has advantages for which it is designed, however, each can have a disadvantage as well. One type of filling material, intended to be used with a root canal tooth, draws moisture from the tooth. It was not made to be used on a vital (living) tooth. If it is used on a vital tooth, it will also draw moisture from that tooth and, in effect, cause it to become very sensitive and most likely die. Since you will not know the difference, have your dentist explain what type of temporary filling material is being used. If you do not want an explanation, just ask for one that contains eugenol if your tooth is alive and you should be OK. You can smell the eugenol when it is placed into your tooth, you may even taste it.

SILVER FILLINGS

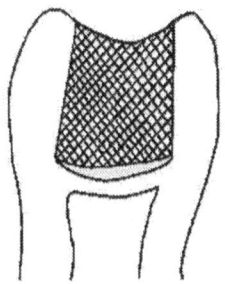

Silver fillings are the most common type of fillings. They are very strong and durable. It is still one of the best filling material we have available.

Silver fillings have been around for a long time and have improved over the years. Most people who have fillings will have some of this type. I'll give you some things to watch for if you have silver fillings or if you need silver fillings. Let's no longer call them silver fillings. They are called alloys, or amalgams. I'll call them alloys.

There are different types of alloys, each with its own properties. If you see one dentist, they may use one type and another dentist will use something different. It is unreasonable to expect the same result from both. Alloys are like cars. You have different qualities in each. You have different things one alloy will do well, while another will do something else. You have cheap alloys and better, more expensive alloys. It does not hurt to ask your dentist which type they are using and why.

When speaking about fillings you must, I repeat, must keep in mind that each filling is unique. There are variables associated with each tooth. You will not have the exact same results with all of them.

When an alloy is placed into your tooth, request that the dentist who places it place a base or insulator under the alloy. The reason is if the cavity had any depth at all, your tooth is going to be sensitive to hot and cold. This can continue for up to a year and maybe longer. This is because the alloy is a conductor of temperature to the nerve of the tooth. If a thick base is applied, it can cut down on sensitivity because it acts as a barrier between the nerve and the filling. However, to much base will decreases the depth of the alloy, increasing the chance that the alloy will fracture. You have to trust your dentist about how thick of a base to have. However, ask for some base, a little protection is better than none.

If you have tight contacts between your teeth. You should expect the dentist to restore tight contacts when they place a filling into your mouth. If your teeth have open contacts or wide spaces, don't expect the dentist to close the space. If the space is small, maybe they can. However, if the space is large and they fill it in, you run the risk of the filling breaking because you will have unsupported alloy.

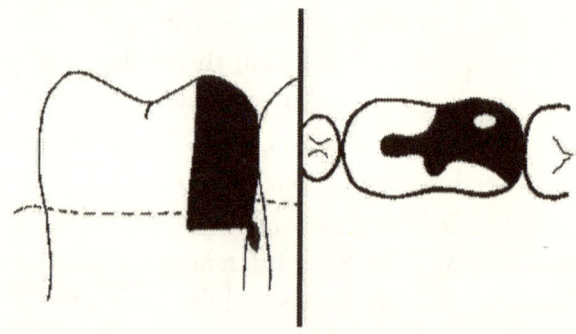

A small amount of alloy may be formed below the margins of a tooth. It is called an overhang. It is very important that this be removed. If left in your mouth, it will trap debris and bacteria and be the starting place for decay and gum disease.
A high spot on a filling (or a crown) will appear as a very shiny spot.

It may be very small in size, but you must have it removed when you notice it. To neglect it could mean additional and very expensive dental work.

On occasion, when an alloy is placed, the dentist will leave what is called an overhang. It is a small outcrop of alloy located at the bottom of the filling; below the gum line. If this overhang is left on your tooth, it will trap bacteria and acids that will attack your teeth and gums. There should be no overhang. The dentist should run floss between your teeth before they finish. If the floss catches, there is an overhang. They should remove it right then. It will take additional time, but it is very important to your dental health to have it removed. You deserve to have it done right.

The result of leaving an overhang is you cannot properly clean under it and sometimes even between your teeth. This also contributes to the development of gum disease, bone loss, and more cavities. Get the overhang removed before you leave the office. If you notice it after you leave the office, go back and have it removed as soon as you can. There should be no charge if that dentist is the one who did the filling. Whenever you have X-rays taken of your teeth, look at them yourself and have the dentist point out any overhangs or any other things that may be wrong with your teeth.

Another thing you should watch for with a new filling is something called a high spot. On new, and sometimes even old fillings, it will show up as a shiny spot. If you notice one, it means you are hitting that small spot before the rest of your teeth are coming into contact. If you have a shiny spot, return to your dentist as soon as possible and have it removed. There are two reasons for having this done. First, so you don't break out the filling. Second, as you keep hitting this tooth, you are causing trauma to the nerve. The tooth will only take a certain amount of trauma before it dies. If it dies, you may go through a lot of pain. You are also looking at a root canal, a crown, or needing that tooth pulled. This can possibly be avoided by having the high spot removed when it is noticed. It is painless to remove and can be done in a couple of minutes.

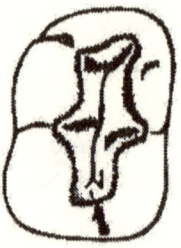 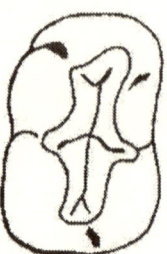

The filling on the left has margins that have expanded and are tarnished. These break off easier and will lead to more decay. The filling on the right has been polished and the margins will not expand much. This filling will last longer and not break down as easy.

Another thing to consider if you have alloys is to have them polished. It is done on a subsequent (another) visit, usually 1 to 4 weeks later. The advantage in having your fillings polished is they will last you longer and do not break down as easily. When done correctly, they will be very smooth and shiny and look like a gold crown or inlay, except they will be silver. Be sure when they are polishing your fillings, they do not speed up the hand piece really high and put a lot of pressure on the filling at the same time. This can create a lot of friction and heat. The results could be a dead nerve and the need for a root canal and crown. I've had all of my fillings polished. They wear and feel better and I want them to last as long as possible. I do not like having them replaced.

There has been a great improvement in recent years concerning alloys. It is called amalgam bonding. It is a procedure that bonds alloys together and alloys to dentin and enamel. The advantage is if you break off a piece of tooth or alloy, you don't need to have the whole alloy removed and replaced if there is no decay present. With the older method, each time you have an alloy replaced, you would lose some of your tooth structure. You can't do that too many times, or you will be wearing crowns. The bonding system allows you to have your tooth repaired without any loss, or minimal loss, of tooth structure. Perhaps the biggest advantage of amalgam bonding is it can eliminate the leakage around the fillings that you now get. In some types of fillings, it will even strengthen the natural tooth structure. It also seals the inside of the tooth and cuts down on the sensitivity with little or no base added. This allows the dentist to place the maximum amount of alloy into the filling, reducing the chances the filling will fracture. It can possibly eliminate the need to have pins put in your teeth to support and give retention to your fillings.

All the advantages of using amalgam bonding are not fully studied yet. It will do a lot of neat things for you. However, your dentist may not be using it. Many dentists like to wait a few years to see what the long-term effects will be. If you think you want to try it, ask them for it before they begin working on you. Also, you'll most likely have to pay extra for it.

There has been a lot said about the use of mercury in the dental alloys. There has been a big effort by some to scare people into thinking the mercury is harmful to them and they must get the alloy fillings replaced with composites, ceramics or even crowns. One dentist I talked with on this subject said that dental alloys were still the best restorative material we have at present, and the likelihood it will harm anyone is very slight. There are those who will have a genuine allergy to the mercury, but they will be very few. He said in some states it is against the law to talk patients into replacing their alloy fillings with other types, unless the patient truly has an allergy to the mercury. I don't profess to know the answers on this issue, but I think it is worth mentioning so you will be aware that the potential may be there if you have an allergy. If it is not there, there is no need to replace your fillings unless they need it for some other reason.

COMPOSITE RESTORATIONS

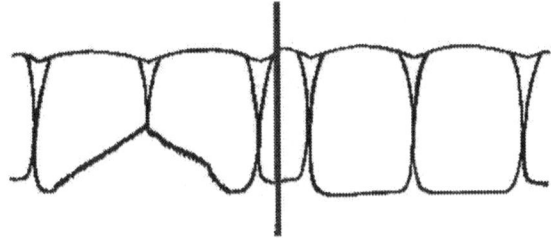

The loss of a portion of a front tooth is unsightly and possibly painful. Have the tooth fixed as soon as possible to prevent additional problems. By using a composite material, your dentist can restore the portion of tooth you have lost. Many times the color of your tooth can be matched so well it cannot be detected.

The term composite restorations may be unfamiliar to you. It is the tooth colored filling material used on our front teeth, rather than using silver or gold. It has been a blessing to all of us who have lost a portion of our front teeth.

There are two types of composites: self-cured and light-cured. The self-cured comes as two pastes that are mixed together. After they are mixed, the dentist has 2 to 3 minutes to place it onto the patient's tooth before it is hard. After it sets up, the dentist will shape it and polish it. The light-cured is a single paste that is placed onto the tooth and shaped. It then has an ultraviolet light placed on it that activates the material and makes it hard. The filling material is then finished to resemble your natural teeth. A word of caution, if you have the light used on your teeth, don't look directly at it. It has the potential to cause eye damage.

There are different sizes of particles in the composite materials, this determines how hard they will be and how well they will polish.. Your dentist should select one that is appropriate for the type of restoration you need. You may ask your dentist why they have selected a certain type for you.

There is also a technique called acid etching and bonding. A solution of phosphoric acid is used first on the teeth to etch them, then a composite resin is applied before the composite is placed. This bonds the composite to the enamel and dentin. This technique has the advantage that little, if any, of your healthy tooth structure has to be removed, as is done when mechanical retention is needed. Another advantage of bonding is there are no margins between the natural tooth and the filling material. They are bonded or welded together. This bonding helps eliminate fillings falling out so easily.

This technique has the advantage of allowing other cosmetic applications to be done such as narrowing spaces between your teeth, covering surfaces that are broken, chipped, or worn, and covering badly stained teeth. The thing to remember in all these types of restorations is you cannot bite hard things like hard candy or ice. It may break your fillings out, so be careful. The composite will also stain if you do not take good care of it. The things that will stain it the fastest are: tobacco, coffee, tea, and certain types of juices. If you want to retain its nice appearance, you'll have to take care of it.

There are many brands of composite on the market. Some are better than others for one thing, but not for other things. It is hard to get one, which will do it all. Some brands come in many shades that the dentist can try to match with your teeth. Some come in only one shade. Don't be afraid to talk with your dentist and know what you are receiving and why. Generally, the ones with several shades cost more. However, the dentist may have a fixed price for composites, so get what you want.

Watch your gum tissue around the teeth worked on. If the dentist does not contour and polish the material right, you will have a food trap. This may be an overhang (see overhangs in the section on silver fillings) or just a rough filling. Test it with floss. If it catches, you have a problem. This can lead to gum infection and all its associated problems. Catch it quickly and return to your dentist. If they put it in, they should correct it at no cost.

ABSCESS

One of the terms used in dentistry that puts fear and pain into the minds of patients is Abscess. How do you know you have an abscess? You'll have pain! There is always pain. It is intensified when you tap with something solid on the top of your tooth or try to eat. You may notice pus around your teeth, and a foul taste and odor.

There are basically two types of abscesses: periapical and periodontal. A periapical abscess will form at the end of a tooth (the apex). It will affect the bone and, if not treated right away, can destroy large portions of bone, which supports the tooth. It will also affect the pulp or nerve of a tooth. It usually means it has or will die.

The periodontal abscess affects the soft tissues around the teeth. It will also result in the loss of soft tissue and, if not corrected, the loss of bone support. This is treated by first having your teeth cleaned by a dentist or hygienist. You may be given antibiotics. This abscess may be caused by getting something wedged down deep between your teeth or under your gum tissue. I have seen this type caused by pieces of toothpicks and popcorn hulls. If you feel pain around your teeth, try using your dental floss and see what you can remove. Be very careful. If the pain persists, see your dentist.

If you have a periapical abscess, you have 3 choices you can make. The first is to ignore it. However, it will not go away. What it may do is form a fistula through the bone and soft tissue. This is a drainage hole that the body creates. It will result in a release of pressure from the abscess and consequently, some relief from pain. It allows the pus from the infection to drain directly into your mouth. You may be able to taste or smell it.

Although the pain is relieved, it will continue to destroy bone and tissue until the source of the infection is removed. If allowed to continue for a long period of time, it increases the possibility that your overall health will be affected.

The second choice is to have a root canal done. This removes the nerves of the affected tooth and enables it to be saved. You will also eliminate the pain you were having. It is suggested you be on antibiotics for several days before your root canal is started. This will eliminate or greatly lessen any pain you may have during the root canal procedure.

The third choice is to have the affected tooth extracted, you then deal with all the problems that brings. In all cases, antibiotics are given to clear up the infection.

ROOT CANALS

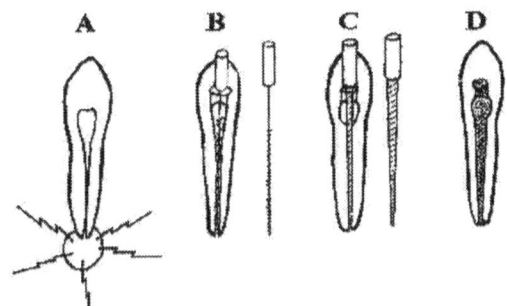

The following steps are taken when a root canal is needed. (A.) The tooth has abscessed. (B.) The nerve is removed from the pulp chamber with an instrument called a broach. (C.) The pulp chamber is cleaned out using a series of different sized files. (D.) After the needed size is obtained, the pulp chamber is filled with gutta-percha to seal off the chamber. A filling is placed over the gutta-percha.

I don't know of any dental procedure that brings fear to patients more than hearing they need a root canal. We all know someone who had the worst pain of his or her lives when a root canal was done. May I say that all root canals are not painful. Many are done without anesthetic and without pain. There are different reasons why a tooth would need a root canal. It depends on these reasons whether or not it will be painful. It will also depend on the urgency with which the root canal must be done.

I will give you a few possibilities of why a root canal is necessary. Sometime during your life you may have been hit in the mouth. It could have been a fall, a car accident, a sporting accident, or a fight with someone, almost any reason. The point is, you took a hard blow to your teeth. Depending on how hard the blow was, and your general health, you could have problems right away or wait for years. It usually begins with a change of color in your tooth. This can range from dark yellow or brown to dark gray or black. You may not have any discomfort. The change of color is a good indication your tooth has died. If it has, you need to consider a root canal. This does not mean you need a root canal right away. You can go for years without any pain. What you may not know is your tooth/teeth will become brittle as time goes on. This increases your possibility of a fracture on that tooth. All teeth that have died will become brittle over time. One thing you can do is have your dentist take your tooth, or as many teeth as necessary, out of occlusion so you are not biting as hard on them.

If you don't mind the color of your tooth/teeth, you can wait. If the color bothers you, then you need a root canal done before you have any other treatment, such as a bleaching or crown. The reason is you cannot change the color of the tooth by doing a vital (alive) bleaching. To bleach it, you access the inside of the tooth. To do that, you must clean out the pulp chamber and canal, or in other words do the root canal. Another option is to have a crown done. However, if you have not had the root canal done, the tooth can still abscess on you. Then you have to drill a hole through your crown to do the root canal. This can give you related problems with your crown.

I've had two root canals and the dentist who did one of my root canals had me wait a year before my crown was put on. This was to make sure my root canal was going to work. Because all root canals are not successful. I thought that was a good idea. If the root canal didn't work, I would have had the tooth pulled and wasted a lot of money on a crown. You can only wait like that if you have a full sized tooth to function with. If you only have a part of a tooth, you need what is called a crown buildup and then the crown put on that. This should not be delayed because you need the space maintained so your other teeth do not drift.

Another common cause for needing a root canal is you have allowed decay to enter the pulp chamber. This can be prevented by seeing your dentist regularly and having your teeth X-rayed. If you haven't seen your dentist, you may notice it yourself if you have a constant pain that never goes away or you can see a lot of decay in your tooth. There are countless ways for decay to enter the pulp. Once it does, if it is extensive enough, you have two choices. Pull the tooth, or get a root canal. If you leave it, the tooth will decay and break apart, most likely abscessing and destroying bone and tissue around it. In short, it will give you a lot of pain and misery until you have it pulled.

When you have an accident and have your tooth broken at a level that involves the pulp chamber, you also have only the two mentioned choices. In this situation, you usually can't put your choices off.

Another cause of trauma that can result in the need for a root canal is if you have a high spot on your fillings or crowns. You can kill the nerve in one of the involved teeth and not know you are doing it. This is caused by the constant pounding it goes through when you eat or close your mouth. It is very important to have the high spot removed when you notice it so you can perhaps avoid killing the nerve.

These are a few of the reasons commonly seen that result in needing a root canal. All of these will not result in painful root canals. For the tooth that has died and changed color, there is usually no pain at all. For the others, your dentist will numb up your tooth enough so you should not have any pain either. The only exception, usually, is a tooth that has abscessed and a root canal needs to be done right away. Please understand it is hard to get an abscessed tooth completely numb. If your dentist can give you some antibiotics for a few days, preferably a week, your abscess should go away and they can then get your tooth completely numb. This will allow you to have a relatively painless root canal. A word of caution, many patients after receiving their antibiotics and having the pain go away in a few days, think they can now get by without the root canal. **This is a bad idea!** It will come back, and continue doing so, until you have the root canal done. It is one of the reasons the dentist will often begin a root canal on an abscessed tooth when you first see them. It is more painful, but it does get the root canal started. If you can commit to returning in a few days, it is far less painful to get the antibiotics and then come back to start the root canal.

You may need a root canal and not know it. The reason is you can have a tooth with an abscess that is not giving you pain. There are usually two reasons for this. The first is you have decay or some other reason that there is an opening into the pulp chamber. This may allow the pus, to drain through the pulp canal into your mouth. The second is for the tooth to form what is called a fistula. This is a small canal or opening between the abscess and the soft tissue of the mouth. It goes through the bone and soft tissue. It will allow the pus from the abscess to drain into your mouth. Either way, because the pus can drain, you do not have the pain you would otherwise have. However, you do have the pus draining into your mouth, which you usually swallow. Over a period of time, this can affect your overall health and the way you feel. If these openings get plugged up, you will get the pressure to build up and have the associated pain. Keep a good watch on any tooth you suspect of having an abscess and get it checked as soon as possible.

When you get a root canal, the root canal will be cleaned out with sterile instruments called broaches and files. Many dentists now use electronic devices that clean out the canal much faster. The cleaning out of the canals may take several appointments depending on the condition and the teeth involved. It is then filled with a filling material called gutta-percha. It is a soft material that can be condensed into the cleaned canal and seal the canal off. In the past, dentists used what is called silver points. They would work well sometimes, but the success rate was not nearly as good as when gutta-percha is used. Most dentists are currently using the gutta-percha.

My last word on root canals is to remember your teeth will become brittle after you have one. You will eventually need a crown. Also, have your tooth/teeth checked to see if you have a good bone level of support around your teeth. If you don't have the bone support, don't even consider the root canal, because you won't be able to keep the tooth anyway. Remember that as much as they try, every root canal is not successful. Some do fail and then more extensive treatment is needed or the tooth has to be pulled.

TEETH WHITENERS AND BLEACHING

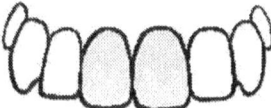

Everyone wants white, beautiful teeth and there are many products that will help you have them. Many you can apply yourself. If you do not achieve the results you want, see your dentist, do not give up.

Both of these terms have the same effect, to make your teeth whiter and more attractive, so I will discuss them together.

I have done a lot of bleachings and I've seen some excellent results. My recommendation is when you have your teeth bleached, you do it in a dental office and under controlled conditions. The dentist may use a rubber dam on your teeth that will isolate the teeth and protect your gums and other soft tissues.

Most of the bleachings I did, were done using a mixture which was activated with heat. This mixture worked on vital (alive) and non-vital (dead) teeth. For vital teeth, the mixture was placed on the teeth/tooth and then heat was applied either with a hot instrument or a light, which generated heat. This type of treatment usually took several visits. For non-vital teeth (a tooth with a root canal), there is a technique called a walking bleach. The mixture is placed into the pulp chamber and left for up to 7 days. When you return to the dentist, they remove the mixture and if the desired results are met, they place a filling in the tooth. If the results are not what you want, they will do it again. We bleached the tooth to a point that was just slightly lighter (whiter) than the adjacent teeth, because it would darken up a little after we were finished.

There has been some controversy about self-applied tooth whiteners for years. I understand the problems were that not only were the results temporary, but you could end up with very sensitive teeth and damage to your gum tissue. There are many new self-applying whitening products on the market that I do not have experience with, but a word of caution, follow your directions closely. You can easily damage your teeth and gums. If you notice any pain or change in the condition of your teeth or gums, stop using the product. A recent article I read implied that in a survey of patients who used the self-applied whiteners, approximately 50% of them experienced increased sensitivity to their teeth. If your teeth start to get sensitive, stop using the product. White teeth that are painful are of no advantage. My recommendation is, if you can afford it, have a dentist give you the whitening treatment. They have access to products you don't, and they can closely follow instructions while protecting your teeth and gums.

Many of us do not have teeth that are the color we want them to be, because they are stained. We all want white teeth. However, ours are usually shades from light yellow to dark brown or gray. You may not believe me, but many people do not have naturally white teeth. Most of us have a slight discoloration in our teeth. It is usually not noticed unless the color is darker.

There are several causes for the stains. One is because of the antibiotic called Tetracycline. If Tetracycline is administered between the second trimester of pregnancy to the approximate age of 8, it can result in permanent discoloration of the teeth. This color can range from a light yellow or gray to a dark gray or blue.

Another common stain is known as fluorosis. Fluorosis occurs when excessive amounts of fluoride are ingested (taken internally), during the same period of time as mentioned above. This will usually happen in areas where the water is naturally too high in fluoride content. The recommended amount is one part per million. The severity of the stain, which can range from minor to severe brown, will depend on how much fluoride was actually ingested.

In both of the above types of staining, the recommended treatment is to have the teeth bleached by a dentist, or have the teeth covered with a veneer. These forms of treatment are very good, but keep in mind that they will possibly need follow-up. The bleaching will last a long time, but usually not forever and the veneers could be knocked off and need replacement. There is hope for those who want the veneers, and that is with the new bonding materials. Some of these will keep the veneers on for many years. A full crown is the closest form of permanent treatment, but do consider that you may be cutting down a healthy tooth and ending up with other problems. This treatment should be considered only as a last resort.

Other types of stain are caused by what we put into our mouths. Such things as tobacco, coffee, tea, and some types of foods and juices will stain our teeth. Most of these stains can be removed by a hygienist or by having your teeth bleached. After you have the stains removed, you will get them back unless you give up whatever it was that caused the stains. Keeping your teeth clean is the best way to reduce the amount of stain you get.

TOOTH ABRASION AND EROSION

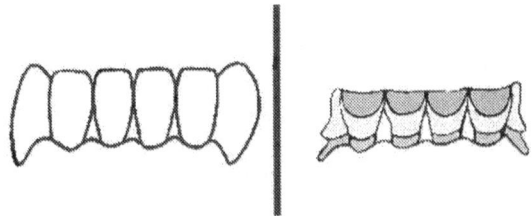

The teeth on the left represent normal teeth. The teeth on the right represent teeth that have large areas missing due to erosion or abrasion. Teeth in this condition may not have any pain. As this nears the pulp chamber you increase your chances of having pain and having the teeth fracture.

If you look at your teeth and notice a groove cut into your teeth along the gum line, or your teeth are showing a great deal of wear on the front side. You need to read the following.

This condition is caused by a combination of several things. Any toothpaste that is to abrasive will tend to wear down the teeth. Using a hard toothbrush can be a big contributor. If you are doing both of these things and brushing incorrectly, you're almost guaranteed to have this problem. Another cause is to much contact with acid or a food with a lot of acid.

How do you prevent it? Use a gentle toothpaste in small amounts and a soft toothbrush. You should be doing this anyway. Angle your toothbrush toward the gums and gently, I repeat, gently message your teeth and gums.

Another cause for this condition is eating to many foods or drinks with high acid content. Some of these are sodas, sucking on lemons or eating to many oranges and grapefruit. Some people who are bulimic and vomit frequently may also have this problem. The erosion of the teeth is one of the first indicators of a person who is bulimic and trying to hide it. The stomach acid affects the teeth and the results cannot be hidden.

If your gums have receded, you may get grooves on the root portion of the tooth. They will wear down faster than the crown of the tooth because the roots are softer than the enamel that covers the crown.

If the erosion is extensive enough, the treatment is to have a filling placed in that area. In the past this type of problem would not always be filled because you had to remove good tooth structure in order to place the filling. With the newer bonding techniques, your dentist can bond a filling over the eroded area, with a tooth colored or silver filling material and not have to remove any or very little of your tooth structure. You must be aware that this type of restoration may not last if you do not watch how you eat and take care of your teeth.

You may experience sensitivity with this condition, even before you notice the erosion. That is because you have irritated the gums so much they have receded and exposed the root of the tooth. If this happens quickly, before the teeth adjust, you will notice a lot of sensitivity to hot and cold. When you breathe in air or touch this area, you will have sharp pain that goes away after a while.

Treatment for this type of sensitivity is to use desensitizing toothpaste, along with the proper care mentioned earlier. You can see your dentist who can give you a treatment using a strong fluoride solution, but it is usually a temporary thing. A recent form of treatment, which shows good indications of being longer lasting, is to have the dentist cover the sensitive area with the bonding liquid only, no composite or silver alloy. Early indications for this type of treatment are very promising.

Teeth grinders not only wear down their teeth, but they also put a great deal of pressure on the TMJ (Temporomandibular Joint). This can cause them to have severe pain in the joint area and even lead to severe headaches. For those who grind their teeth it is not as easy to correct. Teeth grinding can be the result of several things, but it is felt that stress is the most common cause. During the day a person can consciously think about it and control it to an extent, but during the night it is a different situation. Most people grind their teeth the hardest while they are asleep. It can be a noisy habit and irritation to those around them. If you have this problem, may I suggest you see your dentist as soon as possible. Your dentist will give you some ideas to help prevent your grinding problem, but they will also suggest that you try to use a devise called a night guard. Impressions are taken of your teeth and the night guard is made specifically for your mouth. Your dentist will make any adjustments necessary so that it will fit comfortably, anyway as comfortable as you can get wearing something in your mouth. It is made of acrylic (usually soft) and inserted over your teeth each night before you go to sleep. You will likely still grind your teeth, but you will be grinding on the night guard and not your teeth. This will prevent the abrasion and wearing down of your teeth. It will often reduce the pain you may be getting in the TMJ area. Some people have even been able to eliminate teeth grinding as a problem after using a night guard so you may want to consider trying one. (Refer to the section on night guards).

BLEEDING GUMS

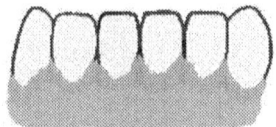

The way bleeding gums are started: Plaque, which is left on the teeth, forms a hard material called tartar. This tartar irritates the gum tissues and they become infected and bleed very easily. They may also become swollen. When the tartar has increased in size the bone structure may also receded away.

Bleeding gums is a prevalent disease and it can run from slight to severe. It usually has the same source, dental plaque. I say usually because there are different medical conditions that may contribute to bleeding gums. If you have bleeding gums, try the things I'm suggesting for a couple of weeks. If your gums do not heal and stop bleeding or at least show improvement, see your dentist or physician for their evaluation. If you have tartar on your teeth, you should see a dentist or hygienist and have it removed. It will act as a trap for bacteria and germs until it is removed.

The best time to get control of bleeding gums is when you first notice it. This will usually be when you are brushing your teeth. The reason they are bleeding is because you are developing a gum infection, called gingivitis. It is nothing to be alarmed about in the beginning stages. It can be controlled and eliminated, and you can do it yourself. If your bleeding problem is isolated to only a few areas, find these areas and be conscientious about keeping them clean. You will not usually develop a gum infection in a mouth that is kept clean.

To clear up this problem, you start by better brushing and flossing. Are you surprised? Don't be. Those of you who brush and floss regularly are usually never bothered with this problem. Refer to the sections on brushing and flossing to see how you can improve on your technique. Don't be surprised when you start flossing if your gums become tender and bleed a little for a few days. This is a common reaction, but you must not give up! After a couple of weeks, you will be happy to see your bleeding problem is going away, if not completely eliminated.

Another thing you can do is use a mouth rinse. There are commercial rinses that may help you, or your dentist can give you a prescription for one, if you have enough of a problem. However, may I suggest something, which may save you some money? One of the best rinses I know of is warm salt water. It doesn't have the flavoring, but it is effective. Just don't make it so salty you get sick using it. Use it about three times during the day. Another rinse is to take a diluted solution of 3% hydrogen peroxide and do the same thing. You must be careful to not make this solution to strong or it can burn your gum tissue and make your problem worse. If diluted (2 to 1), it does a very good job. It can also be used to identify where your gums are bleeding. Use it after brushing and find those areas where you get some foaming action. These are areas you need to give greater attention to when brushing and flossing.

If gingivitis is left alone because it hurts, it will get worse. As it gets worse it progresses to periodontitis. This means it has gone from being a gum problem to one involving the periodontal ligaments and the bone that supports the teeth. You are now in a situation that requires the help of a dentist. The sooner you see them, the less bone destruction you will have. Remember, it will still be a condition that depends on you to clear it up. The dentist will help you, but you have the biggest responsibility. The key is to brush and floss effectively and regularly.

PERIODONTAL DISEASE (GUM DISEASE)

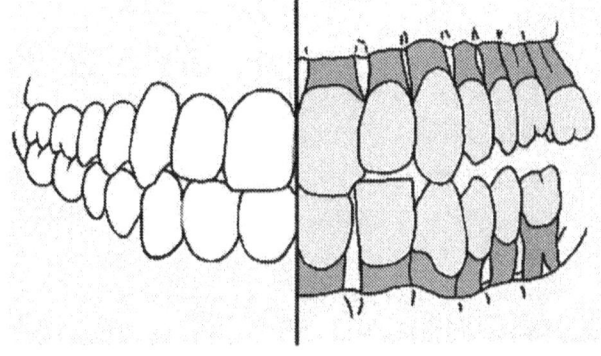

Compare both sides of the mouth. Receding gums are usually a result of neglect. Plaque left on the teeth forms a hard material called tartar. This tartar irritates the gum tissue and it recedes. As the gums recede, the bone will also recede away. The root is exposed and the teeth may become loose and drift out of position. The teeth are very often stained. A very foul odor is usually present. Proper cleaning will keep your teeth and gums healthy.

Many articles have been written about this subject, and yet most people know nothing about it. Almost every person has been affected to some degree with periodontal disease (hereafter called perio). There are many causes for perio disease. Some of these you have limited control over, such as an injury, puberty, pregnancy, mouth breathing and medications such as Dilantin. There are also other reasons, so check with your dentist if you suspect it could be one of these. However, the major cause of perio disease is the neglect of people to keep their teeth free of plaque and tartar.

If your gums are bleeding when you brush your teeth (refer to section on Bleeding Gums), you may have gingivitis, which is perio in a mild stage. At this stage it can easily be treated and cured. All you may have to do is start brushing and flossing correctly. If you do not have a lot of tartar on your teeth, the bleeding should stop within a few weeks. If it doesn't stop, see your dentist right away for an exam. It will likely be treatable with a teeth cleaning by a hygienist.

If you do not treat the bleeding problem, it will get worse. Most people will slack off on their brushing and flossing because it hurts. **Do not do that!** If anything, increase the amount of care given to your gums. Instead of healing your problem, slacking off on home care will make your problem worse. I'm not trying to scare you, but if totally neglected, you risk developing the condition called ANUG (Acute Necrotizing Ulcerative Gingivitis). This is a painful and destructive infection of the gums. It is also a condition, which affects many young adults, stress and being run down are big contributors. Like advanced perio disease, this condition causes you to give off a foul odor from your mouth.

To treat ANUG, you will be given an appointment with your dentist or hygienist for a gross removal of most of your plaque and tartar. This will usually be done with the assistance of an anesthetic because your gums at this stage are very painful. You will be given home cleaning instructions, nutrition counseling, rest instructions, and possibly an antibiotic. It will be necessary to see your dentist again for a more thorough cleaning, when your mouth can handle it better. Don't miss that appointment!

One of the bad things about perio is that it is a slow and painless disease in most cases. Most of us will fit into this category. It can take years of neglect before you will notice any destruction of the bone that supports your teeth. It is surprising to see patients who have no decay, or other dental problems and yet they lose their teeth because of bone loss. The real tragedy is they don't know it until it is sometimes to late. You may have no visible symptoms, no bleeding gums and no pain.

Most will be in their 40 s or 50 s before they find out they have perio disease. They have spent a lifetime taking care of their teeth to prevent decay because that's all they were taught. They should have been taking more care of their gums. When doing this correctly, they also prevent decay.

The way to find out if you have perio is to request your dentist look at your bitewing X-rays for decay and bone loss. Have them show you where your bone level is and explain what you can expect. Also have them check with a perio probe around your teeth. The perio probe is marked with millimeter gradations from 1 to 10 mm, and is carefully inserted between the tooth and gum tissue. Those teeth that are not X-rayed will be checked in this way. Do this each year.

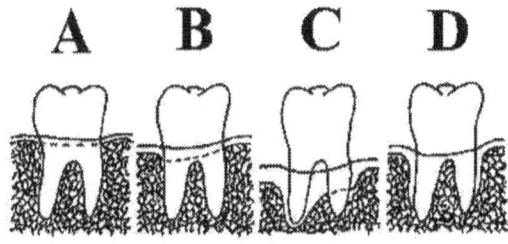

This illustrates the degrees of bone loss. (A) Normal bone. (B) Moderate bone loss, but little loss of gum tissue. (C) Severe bone loss and gum loss. The area between the roots of the tooth may also be exposed. (D) You can also have a deep perio pocket and not lose all the surrounding bone.

The periodontist I worked with considered any bone loss over 3mm in depth to be perio disease. Others may consider anything over 5mm. If you have perio disease there are several ways of treating it, depending on the severity of the disease. If not too involved, you may have it corrected with a teeth scaling and curettage. That is the cleaning away of the tartar and dead tissue from around your teeth. If it is more involved, you may have a perio pocket (a defect down the side of the tooth involving the destruction of the supporting bone). This condition may need a root planing. The tooth is scraped clean and smoothed with hand instruments or a cavitron (ultra sonic cleaner). It may be slightly contoured to remove the dead tissue in the periodontal pocket. This procedure is done with the aid of an anesthetic. This should leave the roots clean and smooth for the growth of secondary cementum and reattachment of the periodontal tissues in some cases.

If your perio condition is more involved, you may need to look at having perio surgery done. There are basically two types: a gingivectomy and a periodontal flap. The gingivectomy is the surgical removal of the soft tissue (your gums). This could include removing the tissue over a pocket and extensive root planing after the walls of the pocket have been cleaned of diseased tissue. Those people who have gum tissue that has grown over their teeth because of medications, will benefit from this type of perio surgery.

The perio flap is the most extensive type of perio treatment. The gum tissue is laid open so the entire tooth, perio pockets and infected bone are all exposed. The teeth are root planed, the pocket is cleaned out and all dead tissue and affected bone is removed. The bone is recontoured and all pointed areas removed. The infected gum tissue is removed. After all this is done, the gum tissue is then sutured (stitched) in place over the bone and a surgical dressing is placed to protect the surgery site. This is left on for about 5-7 days.

This sounds like a painful procedure, but it really isn't. The periodontist I worked with preferred this method of treatment because it was the most thorough. If I ever needed perio surgery, I'd have the flap procedure done. I want to make sure mine is completely taken care of. I don't want seconds if something is missed.

If you are ever in a position to have perio surgery, remember this because it is very important. If you have the surgery done, but do not take proper care of your teeth and gums, you'll soon be back in the same situation, only it will be worse this time. You must, and I cannot emphasize it enough, you must develop a habit of good, proper home care and follow-up with your dentist. Otherwise, don't waste your time and money to go through all that discomfort. Instead, hang in there as long as you want and then get your teeth extracted and get dentures. However, remember proper home care is just thorough brushing and flossing on a daily basis.

People have asked, at which point have they lost too much bone support to consider perio surgery? This will vary with each person and with the type of home care you give your teeth. The rule of thumb is if you have less than 1/3 of your bone support left, it is risky to consider. I have seen people maintain teeth in that situation for long periods of time, so anything is possible.

You may have perio disease in some areas of your mouth and not in others. So, you are not necessarily looking at having your whole mouth treated. Have your dentist give you a treatment plan and explain all that needs to be done.

For those who have AIDS. Often AIDS is diagnosed because of gum disease that does not readily heal after you and your dentist have faithfully done everything you should. Your gum disease may be no different than those without AIDS, but on you it will be manifested more severely and take longer to heal. You must become a fanatic about proper home care. If you suspect you have been exposed to AIDS, have yourself tested.

My last comment on perio disease is that with very few exceptions, it can all be prevented if you start taking proper care of your teeth, dental appliances and gums early enough. There is usually no need for anyone to lose their teeth because of bone loss.

BABY BOTTLE SYNDROME

One of the saddest things to see in a dental office, is when a parent brings in their baby or toddler with baby bottle syndrome or nursing bottle mouth. It is rampant dental decay of the infant's teeth. Sometimes there are no crowns left on the teeth. It occurs when the infant is given a bottle containing a sweetened liquid very frequently. It especially is destructive when either milk or a sweetened liquid is given just before they go to sleep. The sugar in the liquid mixes with the bacteria in the dental plaque and forms the acid that causes the decay. When milk is given before going to sleep, lactic acid is produced which stays on the infant's teeth throughout the night and it continually acts on the teeth to destroy the enamel. You don't have as much of a problem when the child is awake because saliva will help carry the liquid away from the teeth.

If your child must have a bottle when they go to sleep, it is best to give them one that contains only water. Juices can have the same effect as milk or sweetened liquids.

If you are wondering at which age to start brushing your child's teeth, you start before the first tooth erupts. Get them use to having you touch their gums. When the first tooth erupts, start brushing it with a baby toothbrush and no toothpaste, or a baby toothpaste. Brush all the teeth thoroughly at least once a day.

You start using floss on your child when they are older, at least old enough to let you put your fingers into their mouth without bothering them. However, may I suggest using a floss aid, you will both like it much better. If it bothers them a lot, back off. Don't worry about it until they are old enough for you to get their cooperation. Let them watch you brush and floss and they will have a desire to do it as well.

The important thing is to get them into a habit of good oral hygiene at a young age. Your example will be the key.

CARING FOR YOUR
CHILDREN'S TEETH

This area of dentistry could be a complete book all by itself. I will try to give you a few good ideas, which will help you take better care of your children's teeth. As infants, you can start by getting your children use to having you stick your finger into their mouth. Gently massage your child's gum tissue before the first teeth are visible. After the teeth appear, gently brush them daily with a baby's toothbrush. Although toothpaste is not necessary, there are toothpastes, which are made especially for babies. Do not let them get into the habit of swallowing the toothpaste. As soon as they will let you, begin to floss their teeth. If they don't like it, back off until they are older and try again. A floss aid works well with children. Have them watch you, so that brushing and flossing is an acceptable practice.

When children are age 3-4, have them visit a dentist for the first time. It is always best to take them before they develop decay or other dental problems. The first visit can be for a simple cleaning and fluoride treatment and perhaps a sealing if indicated. These are painless procedures and it gives the child a positive experience with the dentist so that they do not fear them. Often most of this will be done by the dentist's staff, with the dentist usually doing the exam. By getting them use to seeing the dentist, they become a friend and are happy to see them. They will not develop the fear, which many of us have. Their first words to the dentist will not be "I hate you", does that sound familiar.

Things you should avoid. Please don't ever threaten your child with going to the dentist or getting a shot in the mouth. They will instantly be afraid and never, no matter how good the dentist and their staff are, trust anyone. They will hate going to the dentist throughout their lives just like many of you do now. They will not get problems taken care of early and will end up having the more extensive treatment done. They will often end up wearing dentures. This can all be avoided by how you introduce them to the dentist. It is up to you.

If your dentist determines that the child does need to have a filling, don't you be alarmed and don't show the fear you may have in your facial expressions. It is best if you don't say anything. Your child will recognize your attitude instantly, trust me. Just let the dentist and their staff handle it. Techniques and dental materials have improved so much over the years, that your child will most likely feel no pain and not have any problem at all. My granddaughter at age 5 was excited to show me the stars (fillings) her dentist put in her teeth, what a neat dentist!

If your child has to have a tooth pulled (extracted), talk with your dentist and see if a space maintainer is necessary (check the section on maintaining the space). If your child develops baby bottle syndrome (extensive decay) see your dentist as soon as you possibly can and follow their guidance to prevent further damage to your child's teeth. As parents of a child, you have the responsibility to help your child learn to take proper care of their teeth, if you don't, who will? Your children will thank you all their lives if you teach them correctly and at a young age.

CROWNS

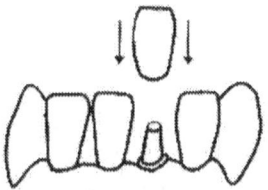

A tooth must be filed down for a crown to be made. Consider very carefully having good healthy teeth filed down, it lasts a lifetime.

There are many reasons for having a crown. Crowns are used to cover teeth that are discolored, broken, misshapen, have had root canals, and badly broken down because of decay. You may have one or all of your teeth crowned.

It appears many dentists will like to do a crown whenever you have lost a cusp (off your back teeth) or a large portion of your front teeth. If you have good insurance or a lot of money, go for it, but you don't necessarily need to. Because of the bonding materials available for alloys and composites, you can have your tooth repaired very well for much less. If you have lost a major portion of your tooth however, you may want to consider having a crown made.

There are differences between dentists in the way they will prepare a tooth for a crown. Some will push the gum tissue back out of the way and prepare the tooth. Because the tissue is numb, you won't feel it. After the numbness goes away it may be sore for a few hours or even a day or so. Some cut the tissue out with the dental burs as they file the tooth down. This will leave the tissue very sore and it will take weeks to heal. Ask before you have a crown done and take the method you prefer.

Crowns are made of gold, ceramic, gold and ceramic, nonprecious metals, and nonprecious metals and ceramic. There is always a debate over nonprecious metals versus gold. You may want to have your dentist explain the differences between the two before you make your decision.

If you are going to have a crown on a front tooth, don't expect it to perfectly match the color of your other teeth. It is hard to match what nature has given you by looking at a tooth shade guide and picking one to match yours. You have a big advantage if your dentist does their own lab work, or if they have a lab technician come and take the color shade. Most dentists send their lab work to another city and that lab can only go by what is written down on the lab prescription form. With your front teeth, the color difference is not so noticeable when several teeth are done at the same time. This depends on the condition of the other teeth, the cost, and how much it is worth to you.

After your crown is inserted, you should be able to use floss without catching the floss on the margins of the crown. If you catch the margins, you may have an overhang. Return to your dentist and have the margins adjusted. The margins that catch floss will also trap bacteria and debris. This will increase the possibility of getting decay under your crown. If you do not want to return to your dentist, be sure you floss and brush under the overhang. If you keep it clean, you lessen the possibility of getting decay. However, you really should consider returning to your dentist and have the overhang removed. You paid to have your tooth fixed correctly, so get it done correctly.

Something for you to consider when having your crown cemented. Talk with your dentist about having your crown bonded on instead of using regular cement. It should not wash out like regular cements do, thereby decreasing the possibility of decay. It is reported to hold better and longer. It is a fairly recent development in dentistry and every dentist may not be using it. Many will give it a few years to prove its worth. If you want it done, talk with your dentist before they begin.

A few words of caution, before you consider having a crown made, know the periodontal condition of your tooth. If your tooth is not likely to last long or needs other extensive treatment, you may want to reconsider the investment. Also, when the dentist is preparing your teeth, request they use a water spray to keep the tooth cooled down and they do not grind off the tooth structure too fast. If a tooth is traumatized too much during this process, you can expect to come back and have a root canal done. That does not mean you still won't end up needing a root canal. Having a crown made may be too much trauma for the tooth.

If you get your crown inserted and leave the dental office, then notice you hit the crown high (hit it before you hit your other teeth). Return immediately, or as soon as you can, and have the crown adjusted. If you continue to bite on this high spot, you risk killing the nerve because of the trauma you are creating. It does not take long to do this damage, a few days could do it. If you kill the nerve, you are looking at a root canal, or having the tooth extracted. That is a lot of additional expense and pain that you can avoid. It will only take a couple of minutes to adjust the crown, and there should be no additional cost.

While I'm talking about crowns, let me mention temporary crowns. They are primarily used as an interim protection device while your teeth are being worked on. They are not designed to last for years, although many do. They are usually made of plastic, stainless steel or aluminum. They are adapted chair side by a dentist or assistant, and cemented in place. The big problem with these is they often have open margins, large overhangs, and break or wear out easily. They can give you long lasting problems if they are left for long periods. Keep the area around them clean. When flossing, do not pull your floss up and down to get it out. Release one end and pull it out. Do not chew on them, if possible. However, if you have to, avoid anything hard. If they break or come loose, get them replaced right away. See your dentist and get them replaced with something permanent as soon as you can.

BRIDGES

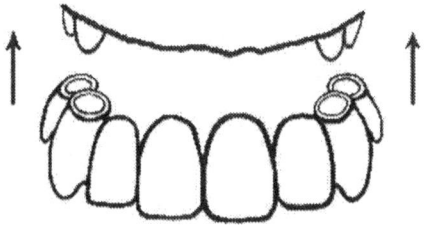

This illustrates an eight-unit bridge. There are two abutment teeth at each end and this will give you much more stability.

A bridge in a person's mouth is similar to a bridge we have all crossed over. It is anchored at each end and has a span in-between. It is different in a person's mouth, the space in-between is filled with something resembling your natural teeth, both in appearance and function.

Before having a bridge made, have the health of the anchor teeth evaluated. If they are involved with extensive periodontal disease, you may want more teeth extracted before you get the bridge. Talk with your dentist and have them show you, on your X-rays, where your current bone level is. Decide after you have an estimate of how long they can be expected to last. Be careful of using any tooth/teeth that are periodontally involved. They usually do not last without having extensive periodontal treatment, and developing a strict program of good oral hygiene. I would be careful when considering using a bridge to stabilize teeth that are periodontally involved. They usually are not successful.

Is a bridge necessary? That depends on the location of the missing tooth/teeth. As a rule, bridges serve several important functions. They help keep the teeth aligned in the mouth. The teeth will tend to drift forward into the empty space where the missing tooth/teeth were located. This can cause malocclusion problems. That means your teeth will not bite the way they did before you lost the other tooth/teeth. Your appearance can be changed by this shifting as well, especially if the tooth is missing from the front of your mouth.

The bridge will prevent the opposing tooth/teeth from doing what is called super erupting. In other words, a tooth will continue to grow and fill in the space on the opposing arch where the missing tooth/teeth were located. It will become longer than the adjacent teeth. This is unsightly, and can cause other problems if left uncorrected. This is why dentists will advise you to replace any missing teeth with some form of false teeth. They will advise you to do this as soon as possible.

You should wait from 3 to 5 weeks after an extraction before you begin work on a bridge. The waiting time is needed because your gum tissue will shrink at the extraction site. If the bridge is made before the shrinkage is completed, you could have an unsightly space under your bridge. This is more critical for the front teeth than the back teeth.

There are several types of bridges and they each serve a special function. I will stick to the most common type, which 90% of us will use. It is anchored at each end by fitting over a tooth, which has been filed down, similar to a tooth prepared for a crown. These are called your anchor or abutment teeth. There is a difference in the preparation of a bridge and a crown in that the anchor teeth must be prepared parallel. That is so the bridge can be slipped on several teeth and cemented. If they are not parallel, the bridge will not slip on and the dentist must do a lot of grinding and adjusting to get it to fit.

If you had a bridge put on and it needed a lot of grinding, there is a possibility the margins of the bridge that fit over the anchor teeth were altered. Have it checked. If you cannot bring your floss down and back up without it catching, then the margins have been compromised. The problem with this is you may now have an opening in the margin. This allows bacteria and acid to enter into a less protected part of your tooth, and decay will progress faster.

You may not notice this condition for years after having your bridge cemented, because the cement itself may fill the space. However, it may wash out over time and then you have the problem to deal with. If you notice this, see your dentist and have it corrected. There are several ways they can treat it. If you catch it quick enough, or have a reasonable dentist, they may not charge you for it, if they made the bridge for you. If they do charge you, pay it, but consider looking elsewhere for further treatment.

If you are replacing four or more teeth, you may want your bridge anchored on two teeth at each end. Realize it will be more expensive, but it will also be more stable. This can make a big difference depending on your anchor teeth and how long and how healthy the roots are. If they are your eye teeth (also called canine or cuspid teeth), you may get by with only one anchor tooth at each end. I say this because you will put a lot of force on your bridge when you bite, and over a period of time you can cause your anchor teeth to become loose. This will possibly result in more extractions, and a new bridge. If you have four anchor teeth, it will be less of a problem.

When your dentist is grinding down your teeth, if they are alive (vital), ask them to use the water spray. This will keep the tooth cooled down and lesson the possibility of killing the nerve.

An important thing to have included in your bridge is an opening at either end and in-between adjacent teeth that is big enough to insert dental floss through. This opening is called a sluice way and should be on every bridge so you can keep them properly cleaned. Although you now have gold or ceramic over your teeth, they still need to be flossed. I have seen countless X-rays of patients who have never flossed under their bridges. They have significant bone loss in that area. Some have lost their anchor teeth to periodontal disease. This has meant they now need a larger bridge. When your dentist inserts your bridge, be sure they show you how to use a floss threader and floss your bridge correctly. It is vital to keep your anchor teeth in good health.

If you lose a porcelain or ceramic facing off of your bridge, it does not mean you need a new bridge. There are new materials that can be bonded to your bridge and still look great. Your dentist should be able to provide it for you with results you like. If they tell you they can't, check around, someone else will.

When you have a porcelain bridge made, get the name of the porcelain used and the color shade, for your records. If you ever have another bridge made, you may or may not want the same shade. If you know what it was, you'll have a better chance of getting what you want.

If your porcelain bridge comes back from the lab and doesn't match your other teeth or is not the shade you want, talk with your dentist. Many things can be done. They can be tinted right in the office sometimes. They can be sent back to the lab and have the shade changed, but this really depends on how close you are to the lab and how good the lab is. The point is, you should like the results, you're paying for it.

FALSE TEETH

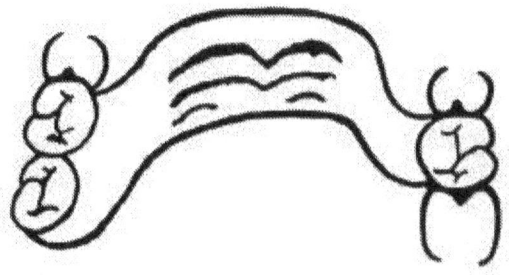

Removable partial dentures serve several functions; they improve appearance, help you chew your food, maintain the space and allow you to keep your remaining teeth. They can last a lifetime if taken care of. You must clean them and your teeth to prevent serious problems.

It is felt by many people that if their parents had dentures, they would also, and they passed that idea on to their children. It has been proven that because your parents or grandparents had dentures, does not mean that you will end up with dentures. If you take care of your teeth, you should be able to break the cycle if you start early enough.

Let's discuss removable partial dentures or RPDs. These are used when part of your teeth in an arch are missing. There are mostly two types of RPDs used today: those made of metal, and those made of acrylic or plastic. The acrylic RPDs are often called flippers and although they can last for years, they are often used as a temporary denture while a metal one is being made or other treatment is being completed. The acrylic RPDs will break easily, so you have to be careful with them. They are not as expensive and can be made in a short time.

The metal RPDs are a more precise partial and more difficult to make. You can expect to see your dentist several times for fittings before they are completed. The advantage with this type of RPD is it will fit better and is much stronger. You also have a wider variety of teeth that can be used.

With either type of RPD you must know one thing. You will most likely experience some rocking motion of your dentures if you have teeth missing only on one side of your mouth. It will be more stable if there are teeth missing on both sides. Your dentist can have clasps put on your denture that will help to hold it in place. However, you may have clasps that show when you smile or open your mouth.

With either type of RPD you must wear it and not leave it out for long periods of time. If you leave it out, you may have your teeth shift. Then your denture will not fit until you have either your teeth or the denture adjusted.

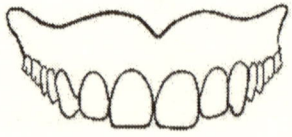

Full dentures can look great and be an improvement to your overall health and self-esteem. Keep them clean and check your gum tissue often for any sores or unusual changes in your gum tissue.

Full dentures, or FDs, will cover your entire arch and replace all your teeth. There are exceptions to this rule. They are when your eye teeth (also called canine or cuspid) are left in place and your FD has two holes in it for those teeth. They will give your denture more stability. These same teeth may also be cut off at the gum line, have root canals done and be filled with alloy. They will then support the FDs and give them more stability.

Expect to visit your dentist several times in order to have a FD made correctly. Your dentist may also make what is called an immediate denture for you. The impressions are taken before your teeth are extracted and the denture is made and then inserted during the same appointment that you have your teeth extracted. You will need to visit your dentist within a few weeks for checkups and a possible reline. This is because your gum tissue will shrink after your extractions.

You will find that after wearing your dentures, the upper denture stays in better than the lower. This is not uncommon. The upper denture is often held in by suction, while the lower denture is often held in only by gravity.

FDs are made of acrylic with either plastic or porcelain teeth. The porcelain teeth look better, last longer and cost more. You can also have fillings done on your denture or have the teeth slightly crooked to present a more realistic appearance.

In discussing RPDs and FDs what I really want to tell you is how to care for them and yourself. Keep them clean and any remaining teeth keep clean as well. When you wear a RPD it creates a food trap and a place for bacteria and plaque to gather. When you wear a RPD that fits too tight, have your dentist adjust it, because it can cause problems with your remaining teeth. If you develop a sore under your denture, take it out when you notice it and have your dentist adjust your denture if needed. For the most part, don't try to adjust it yourself. You can easily make the problem worse, or damage your denture. Also, the sore in your mouth needs to be checked to insure you haven't developed a problem. You should have your dentist check your mouth at least once a year just to ensure you are not developing problems you cannot see or feel.

When you go to sleep, take your denture out, clean it and put it in some water. You should do this every day because the tissue in your mouth needs to breathe in order to stay healthy. It cannot do this if your denture is in all the time. When you clean your denture you can use what ever does the job for you, but be careful using abrasives and bleach. They can damage and change the color of your dentures.

Do not be surprised if you find your denture becoming loose the longer you have it. Often the bone under your gum tissue will absorb or shrink, especially if it is a poor fitting denture. It is vital that you are aware of your bone support under your denture. If you lose too much, you run the risk of needing extensive surgery to rebuild that bone, if in fact it can be rebuilt.

If you find that your dentures are loose and need a lot of adhesive to hold them in, your dentist may be able to help you by doing a denture reline. When your dentures will stay in without any adhesive and are comfortable to wear, then you have a denture that is fitted properly. Anything short of that may need further help from your dentist.

One final comment about dentures. For those of you who wear a metal denture, be aware that your breath may now be more offensive to those around you. People who wear anything like metal dentures and orthodontic appliances may have a breath problem that the rest of the population does not have. Just be aware.

TOOTH SENSITIVITY

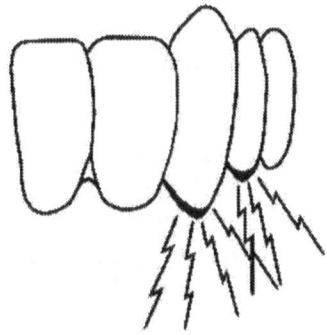

Many who are dedicated to taking care of their teeth develop areas that are very sensitive. Often these areas are near the gum line and, if caught quickly, the sensitivity can be eliminated. It does not mean you have decay because your teeth are sensitive.

Many people have tooth sensitivity and the numbers are growing. It is usually found in people who are trying to take good care of their teeth and are concerned about them. The reason for most of the sensitivity is not what you would think. Would you believe that most of the time, you are doing it to yourself? The most common reasons are brushing your teeth incorrectly, using the wrong type of toothbrush, or using too much of the wrong type of toothpaste. We also tend to brush to hard when we want to remove stains or make our teeth whiter.

If you are brushing wrong, by this I mean doing it to hard with the wrong type of motion, you may have damaged the gum tissue around the teeth. This tissue will then tend to shrink and after a while, it will shrink enough to expose the root of the tooth. If this happens quickly, your teeth will not have a chance to adapt to the loss of the tissue and they will become sensitive to hot and cold, sweets, and even air. If you touch this area with anything, it hurts! You can also remove the outer protective layer on the enamel of your teeth. This is a very thin layer that protects your teeth and keeps them from being so sensitive. Some people who have brushed to hard and removed this layer have teeth that are so sensitive they cannot even breath in cool air through their mouth.

There are treatments that your dentist can do. If no decay is involved, they can give you a fluoride treatment on the sensitive teeth. This is a higher concentration of fluoride and not what is used on children's teeth. Another option is to put on the bonding liquid only which seals the tooth and stops the pain. You'll only be able to get these treatments from your dentist. You will need to change your brushing technique. See the section on brushing and always use a soft toothbrush.

If you are brushing wrong, with the wrong type of toothbrush, you can end up with erosion of your teeth. The more the erosion, the more the possibility of sensitivity. Your dentist may treat erosion by the treatments mentioned above or by putting in a bonded filling. If you have lost any gum tissue, they have a composite filling which is pink to match your gum tissue. If you are brushing your teeth with a hard or medium type of toothbrush, that may be the cause of your sensitivity. I strongly encourage you to try using a soft toothbrush and see if there is a difference. You may need to change your brushing habits so you can avoid needing it done again.

Surprisingly enough, toothpaste is one of the leading causes of tooth sensitivity. Many contain abrasive materials and when used too often or too much, can cause sensitivity to your teeth. We tend to use large amounts of the type that advertise they remove stain and whiten your teeth because we are in a hurry to have our teeth white again and we overdo it. If you use these types of toothpaste, use small amounts and don't overdo the brushing. If your teeth start to get sensitive, continue to brush regularly, but stop using toothpaste for a while and let your teeth recover. Teeth that become very sensitive are a bigger problem than they were when they were not as white as you wanted them to be.

Another cause are the self applied teeth whitening (bleaching) treatments. Each time the acid is applied to your teeth, you break down a very small portion of the enamel of your teeth. If this is done too rapidly or extensively, you can cause your teeth to become sensitive. If this happens, stop applying the whitening treatments for a while and after the sensitivity is gone, then proceed with caution and be aware of what your teeth are telling you.

If you want to stop the sensitivity yourself, try not using any toothpaste at all for a couple of weeks. Brush with only your soft toothbrush and use a warm mouthwash with fluoride to freshen your breath. It will take some time, but it may work and save you a trip to the dentist. If it doesn't work, try a toothpaste that is made for sensitive teeth. It takes using it for a while to get the results you want, and they may not taste as good, but they will ease your sensitivity. If you can find it, try using a fluoride gel instead of toothpaste.

There are other things that cause sensitivity. Chewing hard things like ice, and hard candy can do this. Eating to many foods with high acid content can also contribute (sucking on lemons). With each of these things, it is simply a matter of changing your habits and giving your teeth time to adjust. If the sensitivity does not go away, have your dentist check for a defective filling or a hairline fracture. They are sometimes hard to detect and can be very painful. If you have one, it means having more work done on your teeth.

SCALING (CLEANING) YOUR OWN TEETH

It used to be this was not a problem, but with dental instruments now available to the public, more injuries are happening. It is not impossible to clean your own teeth with a scaling instrument. I do my own, but I'm also a trained hygienist. I'm sure there are many dentists and hygienists that clean their own teeth. If you are not trained, you can hurt yourself or someone else if you try to clean their teeth. You can very easily get an instrument wedged between your teeth and damage them trying to get it out. You can also gouge or scratch the surface of your teeth and cause permanent damage. Perhaps the easiest thing to damage is your gum tissue or the membrane tissue around each tooth. While it will heal in time, you can go through a lot of pain and it could lead to more severe and permanent problems.

If you think you have to clean your teeth, (I strongly discourage you from trying), don't try anything below the gum line and be very careful between your teeth. Some of the damage could cost you more to repair than you will ever save by doing it yourself.

I had a patient who cleaned his teeth with a paper clip. He had very little tartar (calculus) but he did have some bad scratches and grooves on his teeth. He would have been better off seeing a hygienist and then taken good care of his teeth so he would not develop the tartar and stain. You can prevent the tartar and stain completely if you want to. See the sections on brushing and flossing.

TONGUE BRUSHING

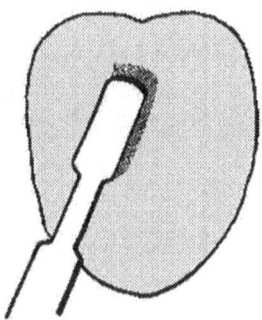

Cleaning the tongue has been done for centuries. It is important and you will notice some worthwhile benefits from doing it.

Brushing your tongue is a practice that has existed for centuries. It was not usually done with a toothbrush. People used a device called a tongue scraper, and they would scrape their tongues with it. You can still purchase tongue scrapers and they still work. However, we are fortunate that we can do it effectively with our toothbrush.

Do you need to brush your tongue? Yes! Your tongue is an area on which bacteria and other materials build up. If you look in a mirror and see a coating on your tongue (usually white) then you'll see what I mean. If this is left on your tongue, it can cut down on your sense of touch and taste. It also aids in causing you to have bad breath.

To get rid of this coating, brush your tongue when you brush your teeth. Brush as far back as the coating goes, or as far back as you can without gagging yourself. With continued effort, you'll be able to brush farther back and it will not bother you as much. Once this coating is removed, you can cut down on the amount of time or the frequency of your brushing, but don't stop completely.

As indicated, one advantage of brushing your tongue is it will help decrease your bad breath problem. It will not eliminate it because there are other contributors to bad breath. Another advantage, and some may not think it is an advantage, you'll be able to taste your food better.

If you have brushed your tongue for a long time (a month or longer) and still have a coating that doesn't change or gets worse, you need to see your dentist and have it evaluated. You may have some problems only they can help you with. Don't put it off!

MAINTAINING THE SPACE

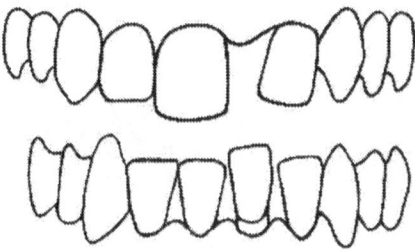

When you lose a front tooth and do not replace it, the other teeth drift forward and fill the space. The opposing tooth will grow into the empty space left when a tooth is extracted and nothing is put there to fill the space.

This is a hard area to write about, because of the many factors that must be considered. However, it is important that you understand the consequences of losing a tooth and what can happen.

When a tooth is extracted (pulled or knocked out), two things happen. One is the teeth behind the one extracted will tend to drift forward. The other is that if enough space is available, the teeth above/below the one extracted will tend to grow into that vacant space.

If your teeth drift forward into the vacant space and the missing tooth was a front tooth, you will alter your normal appearance. It can also throw off your bite. Your front teeth will drift forward easier than your back teeth because they do not lock themselves in naturally. Your back teeth can lock themselves in and may drift very little, if your teeth are not worn flat. When your teeth drift forward, you will need orthodontics to again open the space so a false tooth can be placed.

If you are missing several teeth and do not replace them for some-time with false teeth, you run the risk of having the opposing teeth grow into the vacant space. This can cause you to lose those teeth if you decide later to get a false tooth/teeth because there will be no room left for the false teeth.

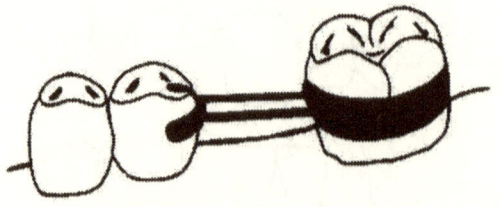

After losing a tooth, if there is some time left before another tooth will grow in, have your dentist place a space maintainer in the vacant space.

If you are still young enough to have teeth that will grow in, have your dentist make a space maintainer for you. This will keep your teeth from drifting and give the tooth space enough to grow in to. If you have all your teeth and lose one of them, have your dentist make you a partial or a bridge. Get something to maintain the space. Don't wait for your teeth to drift and then need orthodontics to move them back, or lose more of them in order to have your teeth fixed. If you do noth-ing, you may pay a heavy price for it later. The odds are really against you.

SEALANTS

Parents may want to look at this closely and consider it for their children. The reason for using a sealant is because the anatomy of the back teeth (molars and bicuspids) is made of high and low places formed by different angles coming together. Where these angles come together in the low places, they create what is called a pit or a fissure. These pits and fissures are often too small to get your toothbrush into. Consequently, you have an area for food and bacteria to form and do their destruction on the enamel of your teeth. This is usually the first area to get decay.

When you notice new teeth coming into the back of your child's mouth, usually 2 to 4 teeth, go to your dentist and have those teeth evaluated for having sealants done. If sealants are done, they will use a technique that will put a composite or resin into those pits and fissures and it will adhere to the tooth. This prevents bacteria from occupying that space and causing decay. The procedure does not take long and is painless. Have it checked each time they are in for a checkup, or at least yearly, because they can be worn off or in rare cases dislodged and need to be replaced.

In the past this procedure could only be done on a tooth that never had decay in it. If you had a filling in the tooth, it didn't work. However, with the advanced technology we have, materials can be bonded to both the enamel and the filling material. So it would still be an advantage for your child to have each of their back teeth sealed. This procedure should be done on your child until they are old enough to develop good, sound hygiene habits that will keep their teeth clean enough to avoid decay.

IMPLANTS

One of the more exciting areas of dentistry is implants and many dentists are eagerly taking training so they can participate in it. It is not, however, a new area of dentistry. It has been around for years, but it has had mixed results, and until recently, mostly unsatisfactory. The problems were that the body would reject the devices that were implanted. You were lucky to get one to last more than a few years.

The good news is there are new materials and techniques which greatly improve the chances for success with implants. I'm not familiar with them to any great extent, so I will not give you any comments on which type to go with. I will say, if you are thinking about implants, you should talk with others who have them and see what their results have been. Find a dentist that has been doing them for a while, or at least one you trust, and have all your questions answered. If they cannot answer all of your questions satisfactorily, go to someone else.

The important thing is, even though you may go for this type of treatment, you must still keep it clean with proper brushing and flossing or you will lose it, just like you can your natural teeth. This type of treatment is not a quick fix to having your teeth replaced. It takes a long time (several months), to have it completed. Find out how long up front and consider everything before you go with it. Good Luck!

MOUTH GUARDS

Many of you will have need of a device called a mouth guard. It is always advised for those who participate in sports, especially contact sports such as boxing, basketball and football. This type can be picked up at sporting goods stores and made at home by following the instructions. Weekend athletes should consider using one.

The other type of mouth guard is used most often for two reasons: teeth grinding and TMJ (Temporomandibular Joint) problems. They may be related because those who grind their teeth, often have TMJ problems.

A mouth guard provides something for teeth grinders to grind on without wearing down their teeth. This can help relieve the sensitivity caused by grinding your teeth. A mouth guard will open your mouth slightly, this can relax the TMJ and thus relieve some of the discomfort in the TMJ. Mouth guards must be kept clean and you should brush and floss before wearing one. They will need to be replaced because they most often are made of a soft resin (plastic) material and can be worn out with the constant grinding.

For a mouth guard used by a tooth grinder or someone with a TMJ problem, you need to see a dentist. They will take an impression of your teeth and have the mouth guard made in a lab. You will usually receive it and have it adjusted at another appointment. It is an excellent way to treat the above problems and should be tried before more extensive and expensive types of treatment are tried.

HOW TO PICK A DENTIST?

This question is often asked, so here are several suggestions you may want to consider. Get your telephone book and see what dentists are available and what specialties are in your area. Get a recommendation from your previous dentist if they know any one in that area. The most widely used method is to ask around. Talk with neighbors, friends, relatives, and associates. If you know any hygienists or dental assistants, ask them. They usually know several dentists in the area and something about the quality of their work.

It is suggested to pick someone who belongs to the American Dental Association, or the State Dental Association. These are good guides, but don't exclude someone because they don't belong. Membership in these associations is expensive and some choose not to pay the added cost. That certainly does not mean they are less qualified or their work does not meet standards. Many very good dentists do not belong. It is not required.

One dentist had the reputation of being the best in town because he had, for the most part a closed practice and took very few new patients. He was also the most expensive dentist in town. Was he the best? That is strictly up to you as a patient. This dentist was good, but so were many others, and they cost less and took new patients. You could also get them to help you in an emergency situation.

Everyone would like to go to a dentist with lots of experience. Well, there is no disputing that experience is valuable. However, every dentist will not start their first practice with years of experience, unless they were in the military or worked for a government agency or HMO. There are some very good new dentists, many of them are more acquainted with the newer methods and materials being used. So if you find a new dentist and feel good about them, give them a chance.

If you are told something by the dentist you picked and it doesn't seem right to you, or you question it. Then do what you would do if a physician told you something and you didn't feel right about it. Get a second opinion. I did with my son, and it saved us having 11 of his teeth filled when they didn't need it. Your experience may not be as drastic, but it doesn't hurt to get a second opinion.

One thing to look for in picking a dentist is how clean their office and treatment rooms are. If they are not cleaned up to your standards, leave. Look at the section on infection control. Don't be misled into thinking that because a dentist has a new office or equipment, that makes them a good dentist. Every dentist can have the same equipment, it depends on how much they want to spend. What counts is what they do to you and what you walk out with. I've had great work done by dentists with older equipment, and I'd go back to them again if I needed to.

Again, remember what I said earlier. You are not locked into one dentist. If there is anything about them or their staff you don't like, then talk with them about it or change dentists. Believe me, if they want you as a patient, they will do their best to keep you happy and satisfied.

DENTAL SPECIALIST

Let me give you a very brief description of the specialists in dentistry. This may help you decide which type you will need if the occasion arises.

Orthodontist: This dentist treats the many types of malocclusions in the mouth. Mostly they will straighten teeth and correct your bite. Many in this specialty will also work with the TMJ (Temporomandibular Joint). For those not aware, this specialist also helps restore self-esteem in people who are ashamed of the way their teeth look. I've seen fantastic work done in this area.

Endodontist: This dentist will primarily perform root canals and related treatments.

Periodontist: This dentist will primarily perform periodontal treatments. This will include root planning, gingivectomies, and full flap procedures with bone reduction, contouring and transplants. They can sometimes help you regenerate some of the bone and soft tissue you have lost.

Prosthodontist: This dentist will primarily be involved with the making of prosthetics (false teeth). This will include the making of crowns, bridges, onlays, inlays, removable partials, and full dentures. Many in this specialty do implants.

Pedodontist: This is a very courageous dentist. This is the one that specializes in the treating of children. They are especially good for children with handicaps. This dentist could set your child's dental attitude for the rest of their lives.

Oral Surgeon: This dentist is the one who gets the difficult work. They do the difficult extractions, the ones that other dentists feel they cannot handle. They repair broken jaws. They also do very sophisticated surgery as well, with the reduction of the upper and lower jaws and repositioning of the teeth and bone. I've seen beautiful work done by these doctors. One did a lot of work on my son after a bad accident. I'll be forever grateful to him. If you ever read this book, thanks Pat!

General Practitioners: This is also a specialty, just as the others, and requires the additional time and training. These dentists receive more in depth training in many areas of dentistry and can work in the specialties to a much greater extent than the regular GPs.

All of these specialists have taken the time, made personal sacrifices, and paid a lot of money for the extended training and education needed for their specialty. In most cases, it is two to four years of training and education beyond dental school. In addition, there are continuing education courses and seminars that they must take to keep their license and be current in their chosen specialty. Believe me, when you need them, you are glad they were willing to make the sacrifices necessary to be where they are. Be ready to pay the higher cost associated with using their expertise and skills. They earned it.

You will also find in your search for a specialist that there are many GPs that will specialize in one or two particular areas. That is, they have a particular interest in this area and have chosen to focus on it along with keeping their general practice. Many are very good at their chosen area, even though they may not be board certified.

ABOUT THE AUTHOR

In 1971, He joined the US Air Force and was given the opportunity to become a dental technician. He took his dental training at Sheppard AFB, Wichita Falls, Texas. After completing the basic course for dental technicians, he was assigned to Fairchild AFB, Washington.

His first assignment at his new base was in the X-ray room. He was lucky to have an excellent instructor. He not only showed him things about X-rays, he helped him develop a positive attitude about dentistry in general. Something he really didn't have at that time. Working in X-ray, he gained an understanding of the destructive processes, which go on in the mouth.

After six months, he was assigned to work with a periodontist. While working with the periodontist he was trained as a dental hygienist. He was now able to see the full spectrum of the periodontal destruction, from its early stages to complete destruction. With this experience he could advise his patients what would happen and what to expect if they did not take proper care of their teeth.

He was assigned to work in a supervisory capacity. That position allowed him to work with other dentists. It was during this period of time that expanded functions dental assistants were assigned to the clinic. These were dental technicians that had received extensive training and were allowed to do expanded functions. He asked them questions about their work and liked what he learned. He applied for the same course and was accepted. Waiting for the course to start, he worked with the finest operative dentist he ever met. This dentist took the time to show him many things about restoring a tooth to its proper function and appearance.

He attended the Dental Assistant (DA) course at Sheppard AFB, Texas. This course taught how to perform the procedures that were considered to be reversible (could be done over again if necessary). The bulk of the training was in the area of restorative dentistry, putting in restorations (fillings), bleaching teeth, taking impressions for crowns, bridges and dentures, seating crowns and bridges, and adjusting dentures. The training also covered root canals, placing sutures (stitches) and surgical dressings.

For five years he worked exclusively doing expanded functions. In 1980, the Air Force officially stopped the Dental Assistant program. Although the school was closed, professional pay stopped and the specialty code taken away, he was allowed to and even encouraged to continue doing expanded functions.

During the next seven years he was assigned to administrative positions and given formal schooling and training in dental hygiene. He continued to work as a hygienist and a Dental Assistant when there was a backlog of patients.

During the last 2 years of military service he was assigned as a First Sergeant, but was granted authorization to work on an emergency basis as a Dental Assistant.

After his military service ended, he worked for seven years with civilian dentists and as an RDA (Registered Dental Assistant) for the California Department of Corrections.

0-595-21699-4

www.ingramcontent.com/pod-product-compliance
Lightning Source LLC
Chambersburg PA
CBHW030853180526
45163CB00004B/1551